W9-AUD-968

THE
3D BODY
REVOLUTION

THE 3D BODY REVOLUTION

THE ULTIMATE WORKOUT + NUTRITION

BLUEPRINT TO GET HEALTHY AND LEAN

ODY
TION

DONALD DRIVER

WITH JON LEVEY

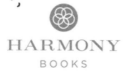

HARMONY
BOOKS

NEW YORK

Copyright © 2017 by Donald Driver

All rights reserved.
Published in the United States by Harmony Books, an imprint of
the Crown Publishing Group, a division of Penguin Random House
LLC, New York.
crownpublishing.com

Harmony Books is a registered trademark, and the Circle colophon
is a trademark of Penguin Random House LLC.

Library of Congress Cataloging-in-Publication Data is available
upon request.

ISBN 978-0-451-49746-8
Ebook ISBN 978-0-451-49777-2

Printed in the United States of America

Book design by Jennifer K. Beal Davis
Interior photographs by Stevan Koye Photography
Jacket design by Jennifer Carrow
Jacket photograph by Scott McDermott

10 9 8 7 6 5 4 3 2 1

First Edition

This book is dedicated to you.

It's never I, it is always we. It is always us, never me.

Happiness begins and ends with you.

Be determined. Get disciplined. Drive to greatness.

#fightforwhatyouwant

CONT

ENTS

THE
3D BODY
REVOLUTION

INTRODUCTION

YOU SEE THAT HANDSOME DEVIL ON THE COVER? He looks pretty good now, but a few years ago he was in danger of becoming just another pudgy, out-of-shape former athlete—a guy who once relied on his body for his livelihood, but when that time passed, he started taking it for granted. I looked at my retirement from pro football as an opportunity to start a new career in easy living. After so many years of a strict diet and intensive training, I felt I had earned the right to kick my feet up and hit cruise control. No more puddles of sweat at the gym; no more denying myself at the dinner table. I thought exercising less and eating more would make me happy.

MAN, WAS I WRONG.

All I became was heavier, softer, and less energized. I quickly realized that when I stopped taking my training seriously, it wasn't just my body that suffered, it was my entire life. I felt like a shell of my former self. The spring in my step was gone. The thousand-watt smile that accompanied me everywhere wasn't nearly as bright. My mind and body—even my soul—felt depressed. I was simply a poorer version of myself.

When you look in the mirror you've got to be content with who you see. It doesn't matter what anyone else thinks—positive or negative—it's only your opinion that counts. After I retired I wasn't satisfied with the guy I was looking at. Because it wasn't me. Not my true self. I had blessings—work I enjoyed; a great, healthy family—but something was missing. I needed a change. I needed to overthrow the lifestyle I had embraced and rediscover the drive, determination, and discipline that had allowed me to flourish and succeed as an athlete.

LET ME TELL YOU A LITTLE STORY OF HOW I ARRIVED AT THE 3D BODY REVOLUTION.

Everyone loves an underdog, and there was no bigger long shot than me. I grew up poor in Texas, and at times I was even homeless, so my future wasn't lined with open doors. My parents divorced when I was two years old, my dad spent time in prison, and my mom was constantly on the move, never letting grass grow beneath her feet. If you judged my prospects based on the accomplishments of the kids who grew up in my neighborhood, let's just say nobody would've bet on my success. And I did my part to buy into the broke black kid narrative: selling drugs and running the street to make it from day to day. People who see the scars on my hands assume they're from my long career in the NFL, but they're actually from punching the windows out of cars before stealing them.

But I realized the road I was going down would eventually lead to a dead end. I vowed not to be limited by my surroundings. I convinced myself that I would find an avenue that would fill my life with opportunity for me and my family. I was driven to find that better path, and I decided it would be paved by football.

Most kids dream of playing professional sports, and I had the advantage of coming from athletes. My father wasn't much in the way of a provider, but the man earned his stripes playing Texas high school football. Legend has it he could throw the ball nearly 80 yards in the air. My mother's family also had its share of local sports stars. I was faster and jumped higher than all my peers—my nickname was "Quickie" because I ran everywhere—so basketball became my first love. It was also the passion of my older brother, and I wanted to do everything he did. But as I got older, and the competition improved, my ordinary ball-handling skills established a ceiling, and football became my best chance at a college scholarship. At that point, the NFL was just a dream. Dreams don't always come true, but no one could take away a great education. I was determined to become the best I could be in the sport—a blur on the field and a beast in the weight room—and to be the first child on my father's side to attend college.

Football managed to take me to Alcorn State University in Lorman, Mississippi. I had gotten a scholarship and the opportunity to show what I could do on the playing field. That was when I first started thinking of my body as a race car—I wanted to make it fast, sleek, and powerful, because even though Alcorn State is a small school, it's part of the Southwestern Athletic Conference, and the SWAC is no joke. To compete at this level I had to bulk up my toothpick-lean 170-pound physique, and I had to do it fast.

Lorman was a country town that didn't even have any fast-food chains. No McDonald's. No KFC. Nothing. Other than the fact that too much sugar rots your teeth, I knew nothing of nutrition. Where I came from, those chain restaurants constituted good eats. So I had to put on weight by turning myself into a human garbage disposal—chips, pizza, ice cream, even gizzard—if it had calories, I was swallowing it. I developed a unique brand of discipline: eat as much as I can, work out as hard as I can. I had poor dietary habits, to be sure—which would catch up with me later—but thanks to a rigorous training schedule and an overactive metabolism, it worked. I was a five-time Athlete of the Year in the conference in both football and track.

My two-sport abilities—I qualified for the 1996 Olympic field trials with a high jump of 7 feet, 6.5 inches—are what made NFL teams curious enough to come to the little, out-of-the-way town to scout me. Of the sixteen, it was the Green Bay Packers who wanted a private workout. Alonzo Highsmith, a former running back in the league, was a first-year scout for the team. He immediately picked up on my desire and enthusiasm. After working out we sat down to talk about my life—where I'd been and where I wanted to go. I told him: "If you pick me, you won't be sorry."

I made good on that promise. Other teams had promised to draft me earlier, but the Packers waited until the seventh round—the 213th pick—of the 1999 NFL draft to call my name. But that didn't deter my belief in myself. It only served as motivation to prove the doubters wrong. There were players who were bigger, stronger, and faster, but nobody could say they worked harder. I had an insatiable desire to succeed. This was what I had dreamed about during those bleak nights of my childhood. I had the drive, discipline, and determination to do whatever it took to make the team and have a lasting career. After playing fourteen seasons, all with the Packers, I retired as the franchise leader in receptions and receiving yards.

But then came February 6, 2013: my retirement ceremony at Lambeau Field in Green Bay. No longer was I required to train every day, eat with a purpose instead of pleasure, and closely monitor my health. If professional athletes are lucky, they play long enough to retire at the age when most people are just starting to hit the prime of their careers. Playing a game for a living was over, and now it was real-life time—three kids, a wife, a busy schedule, traveling and speaking engagements, a return to tasty foods, and less time to spend in the gym. With a packed calendar, I decided to reward myself with a well-earned break from the daily grind of weight lifting and weight watching.

As a result, I worked out less and ate more of the foods I had sworn off—overstuffed hoagies replaced salads, and rich pastas pushed the veggies off my plate. Portion size? What was that? And the thing about bad habits is that they tend to stick around. After breaking my routine of dedicated lifting and making smart food choices seven days a week, I found it exceedingly difficult to get back on that regimen. Those killer abs were now lightly gift wrapped with flab and that 4.45-second 40-yard sprint was a distant memory. Not only did I look puffier, I also felt less vital. I realized that the condition of my body directly affected how I felt and behaved. My body language looked different—no longer moving like a coiled spring—and I didn't feel like myself anymore. When I became soft and full of pollutants, so did my thoughts and actions. Rather than a Pro Bowl player, I had become a practice squad receiver running slow, sloppy routes. My sports-car body was full of dings and dents and seemed to be perpetually stuck in third gear.

It came to a head when I was preparing for a speaking engagement. I was in my house getting dressed, putting on one of my favorite shirts, and I noticed that the buttons were fighting against the fabric. My first reaction was that I had just eaten pizza, pasta, and a caramel brownie with ice cream, and that was why I had the pudge in my stomach.

DENIAL!

Like so many others, I denied that I was out of shape. I lied to myself and searched for excuses. I tried to convince myself that all it would take was for the meal—an excessive meal at that—to work its way through my system and I'd be back to looking like my old football self. But the truth was I had become a cliché—the retired pro athlete who was letting himself go. You've seen those players: they're out of the public eye, only making appearances at halftime of home games to commemorate an anniversary of a championship season. They take shuffle steps across the field, wearing an oversized coat to hide their expanding girth, giving a sheepish wave knowing what the fans are thinking: "Wow, he looks huge. I hardly recognize him."

I REFUSED TO BECOME ONE OF THOSE PLAYERS.

Because I refuse not to be there for my kids and their kids. And I don't just mean alive, I want to be *alive*. I want to be active and vibrant to participate in their lives. I want to walk my daughters down the aisle and toss a football with my grandkids. It's a common desire of people entering middle age, as they realize they may have more years behind them than they do in front of them. Their metabolisms start slowing down, their activity level drops, and things they took for granted—like playing on the floor with kids—become difficult, even painful. I wasn't there yet, but that was the direction I was heading.

Feeling as though I had let myself and my family down, I was motivated to get back to training and eating like an athlete. That was when I felt and performed at my peak—driven, determined, disciplined—and I wanted to feel that way again. When people aspire to look better, athletes are often who they choose to emulate. Bodybuilders have cartoonish muscles, and models often look gaunt and emaciated. But athletes have that lean, powerful, functional physique that is built for life. It gives them strength and confidence in body and mind that they're capable of anything. That's what I wanted to return to, and, as you'll soon read, that's how I designed the 3D Body Revolution for you.

So I went to my friend and trainer, John Simon, and asked him to devise a fitness regimen for me. I had trained with John for years during and after my career, but not as much as I once did. John works with numerous elite athletes at his gym in Dallas. His workouts are demanding but worth the effort. Athletes are super competitive, always trying to test themselves. One of the things I love about John's style of training is that each workout is practically a mini challenge in itself. Every time you hit the gym you're trying to improve an aspect from a previous workout, whether it be number of reps or circuits in an allotted time, amount of weight on the bar, or distance covered. No boring routines based on specific sets and rep ranges. No being a slave to lifting predetermined weights based on a rigid exercise plan. You're constantly moving, listening to and testing your body to see how much you can get out of it.

But a good training program is nothing without the proper accompanying diet, and the truth was my nutritionist was no longer on speed dial. Some people make the mistake of believing that if they're dedicated in the gym, they can afford to be careless with their nutrition. But you'll never outexercise a poor diet. As the saying goes, abs are made in the kitchen. Once again I tapped into the sports world to find an expert in nutrition. Amy Goodson is a board-certified specialist in sports dietetics. She has worked with John Simon off and on since 2006 consulting with pro athletes, endurance race competitors, and everyday exercisers. She also worked for many years as the nutritionist for the Texas Rangers and the Dallas Cowboys. What I love about her approach to nutrition is that it's sensible, it's backed by science, and it can last a lifetime.

What Amy devised for me was not a crazy diet that required supplements and starvation or kept me from eating with my family. This was a meal plan of eating cleaner, more frequent meals, splurging now and then, but first and foremost making sensible food decisions. The reality is that people want a quick fix. They want to lose weight fast and are willing to take risky, temporary shortcuts to get the results. However, if you want a permanent solution and something that will keep you lean, healthy, and feeling great for life, you won't find it in a glamorous, trendy diet. It's eating clean when no one else is looking. It's learning to cook healthfully and shopping for the right groceries. It's choosing a grilled entrée and vegetables at a restaurant when everyone else is having fried chicken. It's skipping the cookies and chips at night while watching TV and being satisfied without dessert. It's discipline. If it were easy, everyone would be doing it. But trust me, you will be richly rewarded for the sacrifices. And before long, it won't feel like any sacrifice at all.

When I put John's program and Amy's nutritional tactics to my own personal test, the results were even better than I had hoped. I started to feel as strong as I did in my playing days with the Packers. The unwanted flab around my midsection began melting away. I enjoyed hitting the gym again and looked forward to each workout. Most important, I got my mojo back. I lost the mental and physical sluggishness that dogged me when I let my fitness slide. I had tons of energy again to chase around my kids and tackle all my projects. Even after hitting forty, I still look like I could put on the pads and catch a fade in the end zone.

Playing for the Packers made me a household name in Wisconsin—and in fantasy football circles—but it was my appearance on *Dancing with the Stars* that heightened my national exposure. If I ever needed to be in tiptop conditioning—shirts were discouraged for many of the numbers—it was for that show. Fortunately, while at the end of my career—I still had a year left in the NFL—I still looked the part. I knew I had some swivel in my hips, but I was surprised as anyone when I won the competition. That notoriety, along with my status as a former pro athlete, later landed me guest appearances as a coach on *The Biggest Loser* and *Extreme Makeover: Weight Loss Edition*. That experience had a huge impact on me.

These contestants were regular people struggling with their health and self-image. Their quest to lose weight was an albatross hanging around their necks, burdening every aspect of their lives. Some endured chronic struggles, while others were once fit and athletic but succumbed to many of the pitfalls of middle age. It dawned on me that if not for the knowledge and opportunities afforded me by my football career, I could easily have ended up in the same spot. I wanted to help these people. I wanted to see them succeed. I got down on the mat and cheered my team through every push-up, exchanged high fives for each pound dropped.

But more than just cheerlead: seing others succeed inspired me to make a bigger commitment. I got back home to Dallas and asked John about getting a stake in his gym. I started taking courses to become a certified trainer. I wanted to be around and learn from people who know the best approaches to health and fitness, and motivate others needing to benefit from that expertise. I felt a strong desire to help people realize that achieving physical wellness will lead to mental and spiritual strength as well.

It kindled a spark to write a book. To quote F. Scott Fitzgerald: "You don't write because you want to say something; you write because you've got something to say." I decided that I would tackle the problem from a holistic approach. It wouldn't be a thirty-day fitness shortcut with impractical guarantees. Your health demands a greater commitment. This would be a lasting lifestyle change. It would not only help people achieve their ultimate fitness goals but raise the overall quality of their lives. This is the book you hold in your hands today.

The 3D Body Revolution is for everybody looking to get in the best shape of their lives—physically and mentally—and stay that way. People new to fitness, those who haven't worked out in years and want to regain some of their youthful form, and even already well-conditioned individuals looking for the edge a former professional athlete can provide will find that this book delivers the motivation and pathway to a healthier, fuller life.

My first goal is to show you ways to improve your mental approach to living a healthy lifestyle, so you can become *Driven* to mentally push past self-imposed barriers and overcome the obstacles and distractions around you to achieve your ultimate physical goals. For many people, the mind will present the tallest hurdle to doing right by their bodies. They don't believe they have the will and commitment to make the sacrifices necessary to improve their fitness. They deem it too costly in both time and money, and meant for the pretty people—not them. So they allow their minds to talk them out of it. They take the easy route of convenience, feeding their bodies too much of something—fried foods, sweets, booze, caffeine—and not giving it enough of something else—exercise, veggies, sleep—resulting in a gaping hole in their health that manifests as a spare tire around their waist and a depressed spirit. You may think poor food choices and a double chin are unrelated to a troubled state of mind, but the two are inextricably linked.

I'm going to show you how to flip that script. I'm going to get you excited and focused on making fitness a top priority in your life. You're going to establish a core motivation to make it so—the inspiration or goal that will keep you dedicated and engaged. Within that broader objective, you're going to create realistic mini objectives to keep you on that path and experiencing success. People want immediate, drastic results and become discouraged when they don't achieve them. But taking smaller, patient, assured steps will eventually lead to great strides.

You'll channel this new drive into your workouts. The exercise plans John and I have devised for you are fun, addicting, and hugely effective. But they will require you to be more *Determined* in the gym than you've ever been in your life. You will need an athlete's mentality of constantly challenging yourself to improve. To push to be better than the person you were the day before. Don't worry if you're out of practice—there are three programs based on fitness level, from absolute novice to seasoned gym rat. The workouts themselves are also easily scalable, allowing for further customization. So you can raise or lower the difficulty on a given day by changing up the exercises or the length of the workout. And as you progress through the program and your work output continually increases, you'll notice that your health and appearance dramatically improve. You won't need a scale to prove it. I can't promise inches melting off your waist, or rippling biceps, but I guarantee a healthier, happier existence. If the human body is like a car, *The 3D Body Revolution* will have yours looking and running like a Porsche.

The next part is to educate you on the importance of your nutrition—don't worry, it's a fun classroom—and how it combines with your workouts to achieve your fitness goals. We're blessed that we have an abundance of food but are cursed with the desire to consume too much of it—especially the bad stuff. Understanding the key components in food and dispelling misconceptions about them is critical in developing an effective approach to eating. This is where you'll learn to be *Disciplined* in your food choices. You'll get the full picture on carbs, proteins, and fats and how to combine them at each meal. The meal plans Amy has helped me devise for this book are based on the same principles she uses with her professional athletes. Just like them, you'll start eating with a purpose: eating meals that will keep you energized and meet your dietary requirements, rather than sheer consumption to appease hunger or a sweet tooth. And I'm not talking about munching on ice cubes and rice cakes, either. These are satisfying and savory meals that are as delectable as they are nutritionally sound. Want to lose weight? Want to pack on muscle? I show you how to eat to achieve whatever your goal may be.

Best of all, it's not a diet—it's a lifestyle. There's no snake oil by way of a fad that works temporarily, if at all. You won't endure radical changes such as eliminating basic macronutrients or entire food groups. You can have the meals on my plan with the entire family, which is hugely important to me. My wife and I try to keep a junk-free home and to limit our kids to sweets on just the weekends and special occasions. I want my family to have the foundations in proper nutrition that I never had. We use the meal plans in this book.

Lock in your commitment to the journey by tracking your progress on social media. Nothing like impressing your friends to keep you going! Tag your post with #3DBodyRevolution to join the community of people changing their health and their lives.

The harmony that will be created within the body by combining challenging exercise with proper nutrition will result in harmony in the rest of your life. It may sound like a tidy affirmation to be stretched across a T-shirt or slapped on a bumper sticker, but the truth is leading a healthy lifestyle and treating the body as a temple reaps far greater rewards than defined pecs or six-pack abs. Sure, those are nice, and aesthetic gains can be hugely important to a person's sense of worth. But the overall impact that healthy living has on every aspect of a person's identity is immeasurable. When you're fitter physically, you're fitter mentally and spiritually. You're better in the boardroom and you're better on the playground. You're simply better.

SOUND GOOD?

Commit yourself to *The 3D Body Revolution*—be *Driven* to envision a health and lifestyle change, *Determined* to take the necessary action to achieve it, and *Disciplined* to never waver in your pursuit—and better is exactly what you'll be.

DRI
FOR C

VEN
HANGE

CHAPTER 1

MENTAL TUNE-UP

The hard is what makes it great. —**A League of Their Own**

As a former professional athlete, I have been lifting weights and working out for most of my life. Barbells, dumbbells, kettlebells, sandbags, medicine balls, suspension trainers, bands, prowlers—if it can be lifted, hoisted, stretched, pushed, or pulled in the pursuit of strength and muscle, I have tried it. Not only that, but I've also had the privilege of working out with some of the smartest coaches and strongest people in the sports world. Massive guys capable of bench-pressing a refrigerator. And after all that trial and error, all that practical experience, I've come to learn one irrefutable fact: more than any muscle, the strongest part of the human body is the mind.

For all its marvels, at its core the human body is essentially weak. Given a choice, it will almost always choose the path of least resistance. The body has to be manipulated and tricked in order to achieve results. That's why we call it training. Because anytime your body is challenged to operate or function outside its comfort zone, it will rebel. Why? Because it's flesh, and flesh enjoys comfort. When the body is truly challenged, pain—either physical or mental—will be involved at some level.

But what I always tell people willing to accept this challenge is this: pain is weakness leaving the body. I love to use inspirational quotes or sayings—some original, some borrowed—that embody great truth in their simplicity. The pages of this book are peppered with many of my favorites. This one about pain is frequently heard at my gym. The body doesn't desire to change or grow because it can be painful.

Because it isn't easy. If it were, we'd all be in perfect shape. In order to achieve a heightened fitness level, your body must undergo a transformation of some sort. The catalyst for this change and the reason you can and will endure any of the challenges presented by my program, and by life, is your mind.

As the mind is composed of your thoughts—whether they be positive or negative—it is a powerful tool. Probably the most powerful tool any person possesses. Thoughts precede actions. The limits we put on ourselves are created by our minds. When I played for the Packers, nobody liked coming to Green Bay. The blustery conditions, snow, and frigid temperatures were extra players on our side of the ball. Southern teams like Tampa Bay or Miami, or domed teams like Detroit—who at one point lost twenty-four consecutive games in Wisconsin—were completely intimidated. You could see it in their eyes. They'd be covered from head to toe and drinking hot soup and we'd psych them out by wearing short sleeves and acting as if it were nothing more than a brisk fall afternoon. Even when those teams were more talented than us, we'd still win. Our minds were our weapons. We beat them because of our will. Whether you think "I can" or "I can't" when presented with the prospect of achieving a goal, you're probably right. And if you're like most people I know, you're probably selling yourself short. I'm betting you're more capable than you think.

When something is difficult, like losing a lot of weight, changing your diet, or elevating your fitness to a higher level, your thoughts are the first to challenge whether it's possible. You look at a picture of a younger you in your twenties and think, "I'll never look like that again." If you allow them, these types of thoughts can dictate and control the outcome before your body ever comes into play. If your mind tells you to quit, or that it can't be done, your body will follow. If your mind tells you to fight and push through, your body will endure the more difficult path. Through mental strength and focus, the mind has the power to will the body past fatigue, pain, and failure. It can override negativity and spur great gains if you let it.

Don't just take my word for it. A study done at Ohio University and published in the *Journal of Neurophysiology* found that subjects actually got stronger by simply thinking intently about exercise. No weights, no movement, just imagery of intense arm flexing for eleven minutes, five times a week. By the sheer force of their minds the subjects increased the size of their biceps. Now, I don't believe you can achieve a healthy lifestyle by simply thinking about it. Dreams don't work unless you do. And my program involves a lot more than just mental sweat. But I want you to realize what an asset mental strength can be. I want you to realize that you can—and will—become driven to achieve your goals.

Because the opposite is equally powerful. I've come across countless people at my gym and on the exercise shows I appeared on who were undermining their fitness efforts with negativity—"I'll never be fit," "I can't eat healthy"—before they even gave themselves a chance. It's just a classic example of allowing their past to adversely impact their future. But what you've been will not determine who you'll be if you're willing to undertake real change. You can't neglect something as critical as improving your health because you're afraid of the challenge. Replacing the negative thoughts you have about your body and well-being with positive emotions and beliefs is a critical first step on your road to better health. Along with it, you need to learn the value of tolerating discomfort and things you don't like to do. And by conquering these minor roadblocks, you'll gain the self-confidence to tackle other hurdles in your life.

Think of all the things in your life that you're proud of. It could be your marriage, your job, your family, or a professional degree. Maybe it's even a skill such as playing an instrument or a material possession like your house. For me, my wife and kids and that Packers uniform I wore for all my years in the NFL are tremendous sources of pride. No matter what you think of, I guarantee it didn't come easy. But I bet you knew that already. Because the greatest successes in our lives take the most sacrifice. Raising kids, growing a career or business, or maintaining a loving relationship are so worthwhile because they also happen to be so demanding. As the saying goes, "If you find a path with no obstacles, it probably doesn't lead anywhere."

The problem is that while many people focus intently on those aspects of their lives, their health takes a backseat. It's seen as something to ignore unless there's a problem. Even if it's severely deteriorated—big gut, high blood pressure, poor conditioning—if it's not broken, there's no point in fixing it. But I believe that if you develop the habits of a healthy lifestyle—working out and eating the right foods—you will be even more successful and happy in those other priorities in your life. A soft, polluted body makes a person less vital; getting in shape promotes self-confidence and empowerment.

Not only will a healthy body strengthen your mind, it literally protects it. Everyone is aware that excessive body fat increases a person's risk of acquiring a host of health problems including heart disease, stroke, cancer, and type 2 diabetes. But an unfit body contaminates the mind as well—and I don't just mean the destructive aspect it has on a person's confidence and sense of worth, which is immeasurable. A study at the Australian National University concluded that the heavier you are, the more your brain shrinks with age. The study found that overweight people had a less voluminous hippocampus, which can lead to memory loss and dementia. Deterioration to this part of the brain also leads to Alzheimer's disease.

But I'm sure you don't need convincing of the value of exercise and healthy eating. What you may need convincing of, however, is that you're capable of enjoying both. And every journey has a beginning. "You don't have to be great to start, but you have to start to be great." It's another quote I love, this one from motivational speaker Zig Ziglar, and it hits at the heart of what prevents most people from achieving their health and fitness goals. The hill to climb seems so steep, the damage you've done to yourself through neglect seems so insurmountable, that there's no point in attempting to change. That's self-sabotage that needs to stop, and your mind needs to be the spark. Research has continually shown the positive effect that exercise has on mental health. I'm going to show you that the reverse is also true.

MAKE FITNESS YOUR NO. 1 PRIORITY

As we get older, we get complacent. We always encourage our kids to be adventurous and expose themselves to new things, but as adults we rarely, if ever, follow the same advice. It's safer and more comfortable to maintain the status quo and coast, even if it's leading down a ruinous path. Nobody goes to bed one night and wakes up 30 pounds heavier the next morning—it took years of inactivity and destructive habits. Interrupting this pattern of behavior calls for bold action that will require getting out of your comfort zone. You're going to have to adopt a new way of life, like the one I'm presenting to you in this book. Psychologists refer to this as embracing a "growth" mind-set instead of "fixed" behavior. And by embracing it, I don't mean trying a few workouts and cooking a few of the meals—people are always dipping their toes in the fitness waters without getting wet. You need to dive all the way in. Be the type of person that when your feet hit the floor in the morning, the devil says, "Oh hell, he's up."

I don't want you to quit your job or move out of the house. Don't miss your kid's ball games or a family wedding. I'm not trying to get you fired or make you a social pariah. But for the time being, make the exercise and eating plans in this book the top priority in your life. It's not being selfish; it's the only way to realize significant change. It will take dedication and sacrifice—in the next chapter we're going to discuss some ways to make it a seamless part of your life—but it will be worth the effort. I don't believe in putting an expiration date on your fitness, but you can establish a block of time—a month or six weeks—to start. I appreciate that having a line in the sand to judge progress can sometimes prove motivating to people. But I'd like you to think of it as a report card, not graduation. Make this kind of commitment to my program and two things will happen:

1. You'll find that the sacrifices aren't nearly as demanding as you envisioned.
2. The results will be so rewarding that you'll have little trouble continuing. In fact, it will be addicting. You'll be astonished that you used to live any other way.

MAKE YOURSELF AN UNBREAKABLE PROMISE

We're constantly living up to promises we make to other people. We vow not to cheat on our spouses or partners and to be there for our kids. We show up to work every day and try to do our jobs to the best of our abilities. I'm even making you a promise with this book. I'm guaranteeing that if you follow the exercise program and nutritional guidelines, not only will you undergo tremendous physical change, but your whole life will improve. If we happen to break one of our promises, we feel awful. If this book doesn't give you the results I'm promising, believe me, I'll feel pretty lousy about it. Nothing is worse than letting someone down. We beat ourselves up and pledge never again.

BUT BREAK A PROMISE TO OURSELVES? NO PROBLEM.

One thing about me you'll discover in this book is that I'm not afraid to deliver some tough love. I don't believe in sugarcoating just to make what I'm telling you easier to swallow. So here's some truth: there will be obstacles. Whether it's struggling with a workout or straying with a stretch of unhealthy meals, there will be times when you're stuck in neutral or even take a step back. After several weeks of weight loss, the scale may point to a number you thought you'd left in your past. Worse yet, you may encounter a daunting personal crisis or professional hurdle. Many people view these obstacles as roadblocks instead of speed bumps. They think it's proof that they don't possess the makeup or discipline to live a healthy lifestyle and use these difficulties as excuses to give up. Don't be that person. Your health is too important. Don't let yourself down by giving up. Make a promise to yourself that you're going to be committed no matter what adversity stands in your way.

When I entered the NFL draft I thought I was going in the fourth round to either Kansas City or San Francisco. Both teams promised me as much. Then I dropped to the seventh round, the twenty-fifth wide receiver taken. I was picked by Green Bay, a city I didn't even know was in Wisconsin. When I arrived that April I got off the plane in shorts and a T-shirt and nearly turned into a Popsicle. I was a Texas kid, a fan of the Oilers and Cowboys, and now I was going to freeze my butt off up north on a team where I was tenth on the depth chart. I felt disrespected. I had plenty of confidence—when asked by a reporter about the weaknesses of my game, I replied, "Nothing"—and now I had the motivation. I came to work every day with a smile on my face and played my hardest, catching every ball thrown my way. My goal was to make it in the NFL. Even after recording only thirty-seven catches in my first three seasons, I wasn't about to let it go. I had to continue to break through barriers to make my dream a reality.

So when you encounter one of these moments—and there will be these moments—you will soldier on. If anything, you should view them as learning experiences. Experience is the hardest kind of teacher—it gives you the test first and the lesson afterward. Because the more times you get up from stumbles, the fewer you will encounter in the future. Remember: there's no such thing as perfect. Whether it's the dedication to and intensity of your training or adherence to the meal plan, it's natural to think you could be doing something better. But better can be the enemy of good. And as long as you're making good, steady progress in improving your health and habits, the rewards you seek will definitely come.

THINK LIKE AN ATHLETE

When you play professional football—or sports at any level, for that matter—positive thinking can be the only state of mind. You not only need belief in your abilities, you must trust that success is almost inevitable. When I lined up across from a tough defensive back like Dante Hall of the Atlanta Falcons, I never thought, *I hope I can get open.* Or if we called a play that I struggled with the last time we ran it, I wouldn't think, *I'd better not mess this up again.* The same way LeBron James would never step to the free-throw line or Serena Williams prepare to serve hoping not to miss, all my thoughts were geared toward running a smooth and effective route and making a play. I'd envision myself exploding off the line after the snap, executing my footwork just as I planned, breaking away from the defender's coverage, and streaking clear into the open field to receive the pass. Or if it was a running play, I could see myself engaging my opponent, grabbing him by the shoulder pads, and driving him back into the secondary to create space for our ball carrier. The ensuing touchdown was inevitable.

I'd love to tell you that all my thoughts became reality: that I always got open, never missed a block, and all our plays resulted in large chunks of yards. But the truth is the opposing defense had players who were pretty good at their jobs, too. They believed just as confidently in their abilities and their schemes to stop us. Dante Hall had no trouble telling me so . . . repeatedly. Things didn't always work out as planned. That's just the nature of sports. That's just the nature of life. So we would huddle up after a failed play, call the next one, and come to the line expecting great things.

I want you to tackle your health with the same attitude. I want you to adopt and become accountable to the same drive, determination, and work ethic. This is what pushes you not just to become a professional athlete, but to reach the top of any profession. No matter what you've felt in the past about your fitness level, no matter what setbacks you've endured, this time is different. You're going to succeed. You're going to be more dedicated and more disciplined than ever before. You're going to drop those unwanted pounds and start feeling and looking more energized. Even if you're satisfied with your current weight but feel stagnant in your current conditioning programs—not gaining strength or putting on lean muscle any longer—you're going to smash through those plateaus. It's not a matter of *if* but *when* you start reaching your goals, only to then reset the bar even higher to scale new heights. Winning a Super Bowl is awesome; a second title even sweeter. This type of attitude will not only help you bring about the lifestyle change you seek, it will permeate other aspects of your life. Work, relationships, and just about anything you set your mind to will benefit from this new sense of confidence. Even if things don't always work out exactly as you envision, you know if you keep at it with a positive frame of mind, it will be only a matter of time.

This self-assurance is also why athletes are so competitive. They love any chance they get to prove themselves. In the Packers weight room we were constantly trying to one-up each other. If someone hit the wide receiver record on the squat rack, I was gunning to beat it. And as you'll discover when you get to the workout programs, I've designed them so that in each session you're competing against your previous best. Whether it's completing a workout in less time than you did before, or doing it with greater resistance, your goal will be to increase your work capacity each time you step into the gym. Keep beating your old personal best scores, and the only thing you'll lose is pounds.

IT WILL WORK . . . TRUST ME

I know what you're thinking: this is all pretty easy for me to say. I'm a former professional athlete and have never struggled with being overweight. Well, as I stated earlier, after retiring from football I did put disciplined eating and working out on the back burner. I can appreciate that when it's not required of you, it's very easy to let yourself go. When you look in the mirror, and the person staring back isn't the best you, it's devastating right down to your soul—doesn't matter if you're 5 or 50 pounds overweight. I also know that when you're on the wrong side of forty, you've got to be smarter about your conditioning. I recognize that my body's metabolism has slowed down and that workouts I used to crush in my playing days could potentially crush me now.

And I also know this may not be the first fitness book you've bought, and the others have let you down. I've spent a great deal of time working with people just like you to discover a long-term solution to leading a healthy lifestyle. I've experimented in the gym on myself, with my coaches, and with everyday people to fine-tune the exercise program. I've worked with aspiring professional athletes, husbands, wives, couples (the gym is a great place to meet someone—it's where I met my wife), even fathers and sons trying to get in shape together. They've all taught me things that I'm going to pass on to you.

You will probably come across an exercise and say to yourself: "I haven't done that since high school." Which should tell you something, because that's when you were probably in your best shape. So often people stop doing things because they think they're "too old" to be doing them, when the real problem could be that not doing them is what's making them feel old. But don't worry—I'm going to help you rediscover your personal best.

Case in point: sprinting. I love to sprint. I ran track throughout college, and when I was an NFL wide receiver, speed was a job requirement. Besides that, though, sprinting is a tremendous workout. Short bursts of intense running are a great lower-body muscle builder and overall fat burner. Yet once people hit a certain age, they wouldn't dream of hitting the field for some sprints. In fact, if you want to get a good laugh, go to your local high school track and try it sometime. All the walkers and slow joggers will look at you like you're bonkers.

So I'm going to ask you to do things that may fall outside your comfort zone. I'm going to want you to incorporate exercises and techniques you may not have ever performed before. I wouldn't be surprised if you even question some of the things I ask of you. Call me crazy if you like. Call me worse. In the middle of a workout my trainees often do. But try not to doubt what I'm offering. Doubt causes hesitancy and indecision. Nobody functions at their best when they're not truly committed. I want you to fully embrace this program, make yourself an unbreakable promise that no matter what obstacles get in your way there is no quit, and believe you will experience the results you seek.

CHAPTER 2
START YOUR ENGINE

If you will it, it is no dream. —Theodor Herzl

How many times have you or someone you know set an immense goal at the start of the new year? Lose 30 pounds, drop a shirt or dress size, add 50 pounds to your bench press. When we first set out, we are full of can-do spirit and motivation. For several weeks, maybe even months, we stay on point in our efforts. But as is often the case we crumble under the enormity of our ambitions. We set out to climb a mountain but become discouraged when it takes more than a few overreaching strides. Our resolve is pummeled by our own resolution.

The truth is that even with the greatest of intentions and the desire to do something amazing, without a sound strategy, we will stumble and ultimately fail. Psychologists have identified six stages of change: precontemplation, contemplation, preparation, action, maintenance, and termination. Jumping right into action without fully embracing the preparatory steps is a recipe for disappointment. For instance, take training for a marathon. You wouldn't start out your first session with a 13-mile run. After the first couple of miles your legs would feel like lead and your lungs would be on fire and it would seem like you're trying to run through mud. Not only would you be discouraged with yourself, but you'd be disheartened with the whole concept—"I'm nowhere near finishing even *half* a marathon!"—and could very well quit.

This happens when you're living in a "Just Do It" universe. Since we were children we've been told to dream big and that nothing can stop us. I agree that having lofty aspirations is inspiring—I'm living proof that anything is possible—but without a practical plan to realize them, these dreams will remain mere fantasies. And when it comes to setting fitness goals, you need to take a deliberate approach. It may seem counterintuitive to start small, but remember that you want to set yourself up for success, not failure. Wanting to go from overweight and sedentary to working out six days a week is an admirable and potentially achievable desire, but starting out with smaller, easier-to-accomplish ambitions is the surest way to get there. The best way I know how is to start with a clear, overarching fitness objective.

WHY ARE YOU DOING THIS?

"I want to lose weight." Ah, old reliable. Without a doubt, that's the pat, ready answer so many people give for starting a new fitness regimen. And while there's nothing overtly wrong with such an ambition, it's not specific enough. You need to zero in on a distinct source of inspiration that compels you each day to be better. For me, it's the prospect of staying active with my children. Every day I see them is a constant reminder that I want to stay vital enough to toss a football with my son, take family ski trips, and know that someday I'll walk my daughters down the aisle on their wedding days. I want to always be able to work out with them, something I have found to be a great family bonding experience. I'd love it if, years from now, I can do the same with my grandkids.

This is obviously different from when I was a younger man. Because of my upbringing, I wasn't sure I even wanted kids. All I wanted to do was a find a way to help my family survive. I remember lying in bed in our Houston apartment with my older brother, Moses, promising him we would have a better life. That we wouldn't have to struggle for money and food, or to worry if we would have a roof over our heads. That meant succeeding in the NFL. When I signed my first big contract with the Packers, I achieved that goal.

Given enough thought and reflection, everyone can discover a definitive reason for wanting to improve their health. Many people harbor a negative self-image because of their poor physical conditioning. The excess weight not only affects their health but also clouds their spirit. For some, it could be that they received some disturbing health news. Mortality can be a sobering wake-up call. I can relate.

When I arrived at my first Packers training camp I was only 5 pounds heavier than when I entered college. I knew that if I was going to stick around, I needed more size to handle the rigors of the pro game. At the time I knew nothing of proper nutrition. When I was growing up, the only thing I knew about food was that we struggled to have enough of it. I turned to the only meal plan I knew for putting on size: gluttony. Every single day after practice for an entire year I would stop at Wendy's and eat two junior cheeseburgers (no onions), large fries, large Dr Pepper, and a large Frosty. I kept seeking out calories anywhere I could. Fat-laden and unhealthy as the food may have been, it did the trick—by my fourth year I was a rock-solid 185 pounds and a staple on the team.

That was the same season the team decided to bring a nutritionist on staff. My dedication to my training was always one of my greatest attributes—few worked harder in the gym—but it turned out that my sloppy eating habits weren't doing my insides any favors. When the Packers team doctor and nutritionist warned me that my blood pressure and cholesterol were too high, it frightened me. Even though there's evidence that dietary cholesterol has a negligible impact on overall blood cholesterol, I knew my habits had to change as I got older. I simply couldn't eat whatever I wanted and expect a middle-aged body to absorb the empty calories like my younger self. I decided I needed to clean up my diet and start thinking about life after football. My wife and I already had one child at the time and hoped to have several more. Staring at the face of your child, wanting to always be there for them, will do more to get your priorities in order than any medical test or doctor's advice.

Others may have performance goals such as improving in a sport by getting stronger or building more endurance. Sometimes less "noble" pursuits can be your inspiration. Vanity is often deemed a sin, but I've also seen it motivate people to make great change. If coveting broader shoulders or looking more attractive in a bathing suit keeps you hitting the gym and eating right, then there's nothing wrong with that. Suck it up, and one day you won't have to suck it in. When something means enough to you, when you're committed to get yourself there, only then will you do it.

So when it comes to setting your fitness and health goals, I want you to be **DRIVEN**.

WHAT DOES THAT MEAN?

DECISIVE—As I stated earlier, you will not be successful, or as successful as you could be, if you adopt a nebulous goal such as "lose weight" or "get stronger." You want to be as specific as possible in your intentions. If you are narrow in your focus, not only will you have a greater likelihood of sticking with the plan, but you'll ultimately achieve the broader goal of heightened physical and mental wellness.

RESEARCHED—Self-help guru Tony Robbins often quips, "Success leaves clues." Learning as much as you can about what you hope to achieve endows you with knowledge and confidence. You're taking an informed step by reading this book. Having a guide and doing preparatory work take away the uncertainty of the road ahead by illuminating your path. But don't stop here; keep searching and discovering in a variety of resources—books, the Internet, experienced trainers. When you broaden your knowledge and learn the most proven, effective ways to achieve your goals, you set yourself up for the ultimate success.

INDIVIDUAL—This is your goal, nobody else's. Don't adopt the wants and feelings of other people. That's a recipe for unhappiness and disappointment, and possibly why you're struggling with weight and body issues in the first place. You need to be happy with the person in the mirror. Look that person in the eye and discover what he or she wants. That's the only way to be happy, and the only way to achieve your goals.

VIABLE—Everyone can get better. But there has to be a measure of truth in what you're trying to accomplish. If you're a high school basketball player with the intentions of improving your work capacity and adding 5 pounds of muscle to your body, those are achievable and realistic. Same goes for someone looking to gradually eliminate 500 calories from his daily food intake. However, a novice lifter aiming to bench-press twice his body weight in six months is setting himself up for failure. When you start to consistently achieve viable goals, what once seemed like the impossible is suddenly in reach.

EMOTIONAL—I'm a passionate guy. And my passion fuels my goals. If I don't feel connected to something, if it doesn't move me, I struggle to give it my full effort. When I strove to make the NFL, I knew what it could mean for me and my family. I worked so hard to succeed and prolong my career because of what it could provide for my wife and kids. It's true that many times pro athletes retire because their bodies fail. But for many the passion and desire leave after a long career, and they're not fully vested in the rigors of the game anymore. Your fitness goal has to mean something to you. It has to inspire you to get out of bed in the morning and hit the gym instead of the snooze button. It has to have the power to fill you with a great sense of accomplishment if you achieve it, and an even greater sense of disappointment if you don't.

NECESSARY—Wanting to add an inch to the circumference of your biceps isn't fundamentally a pointless goal. It's not what I would recommend, but I'm not going to fault a fit, muscular guy for wanting to bust out his shirtsleeves. Improving aesthetic appeal can be inspiring. But for most people looking to strip body fat, improve their nutrition, and achieve an elevated level of fitness, fixating on bigger arms is shortsighted. It's a little like obsessing over the flower bed in front of your house when your roof is leaking. And it's the type of thinking that will limit your success. Because, ultimately, if you don't add an inch to your arms, it's not a big deal. It's a luxury goal that isn't imperative. It's why I bet you know many people with a novel half-finished, or a musical instrument collecting dust. There's nothing sacrificed if they fail. But if you continue to struggle with weight and health problems, those have serious long-term repercussions. The best goals are ones that are essential because those are ones you're most likely to see through.

To that end, it can be valuable to create a symbol of this motivation. I won't insist you do it, but it has been proven effective to take a picture of yourself in your underwear before embarking on a fitness transformation. Then periodically—perhaps every month—you take more photos wearing the exact same clothes. Each time provides an opportunity to judge and be inspired by your progress. Numbers on a scale can often be deceptive, but a mirror tells no lies.

Or, instead of your humble beginnings, you can find an aspirational photo in a magazine or online of someone with the physique you seek. If you're doing this primarily for health reasons, make a copy of your below-average EKG or blood test. Whatever your choice, make that symbol available to yourself—in your wallet, on the bathroom mirror, taped to the wall in your home gym, even as the wallpaper on your phone. Anytime you need a jolt of inspiration, look at it to remember why you're making this sacrifice.

BABY STEPS LEAD TO GIANT STRIDES

Now that you've established your peak—the overarching fitness goal to motivate yourself—you need to create practical and reachable mini goals in order to scale it. When I played for the Packers we were known for scripting our first several offensive possessions. It gave us better efficiency and clarity of purpose. We weren't expecting huge gains on each play, just positive yardage. We knew that if we executed properly and stayed true to the game plan, we'd eventually get in the end zone. First downs = touchdowns. If you try to scale a mountain by leaps and bounds, there's a good chance you'll slip and fall. But if you take small, steady, secured steps, you're much more likely to reach the top.

What do I mean by mini goals? Let's assume you've been largely inactive for many years and are aiming to drop 20 pounds. Over the first month of training, some practical mini goals could be:

- Hitting the gym a minimum of two to three times per week
- Substituting plain coffee and water for Frappuccinos and soda
- Getting 7 to 8 hours of sleep a night

Sure, you could be more ambitious, but I strongly suggest starting slowly. The idea is to build on successes and continually progress toward your ultimate objective. And once you hit these marks—and I bet you lose a few pounds in the process—you can reassess and move the goalposts to create new objectives. A possible second month could include the following:

- Incorporating at least two new movements into your workouts
- Upping water intake to the number of ounces equal to half your body weight in pounds
- Eating some form of protein at each meal

This type of approach encourages steady and effective change. That's why the fitness and nutrition plans in this book are structured in graduating levels. Many fitness programs take a one-size-fits-all approach to the gym and kitchen. This doesn't allow for differing rates of progress or user ability. I've constructed the workouts so that each time you exercise, there's another mini goal to accomplish. It could be simply finishing a previous workout in less time, or squeezing out a few more reps over the same time period. Same goes for the kitchen: you'll continually tweak and improve your diet in a sensible and deliberate manner. As the Chinese proverb states: "Be not afraid of growing slowly, be afraid only of standing still."

That's why it's critical that you appreciate the journey. So many people want immediate gratification and give up when they don't experience it. After a few weeks they're not enjoying the progress they envisioned—undoubtedly due to unrealistic expectations—and start questioning whether the sacrifice is worth it. But if you define your success by everyday victories, the process feels that much more gratifying, and the destination that much more reachable.

Don't be embarrassed or ashamed to pat yourself on the back for showing even the slightest improvement in the gym or on the scale. Take pride in a personal best time in a workout or even a well-prepared meal. Give respect to a day in which you slept well, worked out hard, and ate properly. Those are mini goals worth celebrating. If you're out to dinner with friends and everybody is gorging on beer, wings, and fries but you stick with a chicken breast and baked potato, that's no easy feat. Congratulate yourself on showing great commitment and restraint. Your ability to resist overindulging may not seem like a notable accomplishment at the time, but it's guaranteed to pay off down the road.

NOW IT'S YOUR TURN

This book is the ultimate fitness blueprint. Everything you need for diet and exercise can be mapped out to each meal and workout. Follow the concepts and techniques I've laid out for you, and you will learn how to incorporate exercise and healthy eating into your daily life so it sticks, grows, and multiplies. However, the one thing this book won't do is do it for you. No matter how properly thought out and well devised the goals, if you don't commit to achieving them, they'll be nothing more than pipe dreams.

NOW I'VE HEARD EVERY EXCUSE:

I don't have the time.
I'm too busy with work.
Working out is so boring.
My kids' schedules dominate my days.

My body isn't built for working out.

Everybody in my family is overweight; I've got no shot at being lean.

And on and on. There's no shortage of reasons—cop-outs, really—that people give for avoiding the gym. It's always easier to take the path of least resistance. Sitting on the couch is easier than hitting the weights; eating greasy, fatty foods is easier than preparing a nutritious meal. But even people offering lame excuses and opting to make poor health choices know better. They know they're only fooling themselves. And that's why they're so conflicted. It pains them that they've allowed themselves to get so out of shape, forcing them to erect faulty crutches to create a psychological out. But deep down they know the truth: you can always make exercise and smart food choices a part of your life without disrupting it.

My workouts are quick, designed to last no more than 45 minutes. So we're not talking about a huge time commitment. You can be in and out of the gym in under an hour. Ask yourself: Is it completely out of the question that I could get up earlier in the morning a few days a week to work out? Or if early rising is just not in your nature, or just impossible given family or work commitments, could you get to the gym at the end of the day? Think about what you do from the time you finish work until you go to bed at night: Are there really no opportunities to exercise for less than an hour? Instead of watching first-run broadcasts of your favorite shows, could you record them to watch on your off days from the gym, or on weekends? For one week, write down everything—I mean everything—you do on each day. From when you get up to when you put your head on the pillow. I'm willing to bet that you will find chunks of time in which you're essentially sitting on your butt. You need to turn that time into opportunities to reach your fitness goals.

And please don't keep fooling yourself by thinking you've always got tomorrow. When I was drafted by the Packers, they had just come off back-to-back Super Bowl appearances and had Brett Favre at quarterback, perhaps the best player in the league. I thought I'd be piling up championship rings. But sports—like life—offer no guarantees. It took me twelve seasons and numerous heartbreaking defeats before I made it to that Super Bowl. There were many times I doubted it would ever happen. Nothing is promised. You must take advantage of what you can do today.

The fact is, if you don't make time for it now, you will have to make time for it years from now when your neglect has led to health issues. In 2012, new cases of type 2 diabetes were diagnosed in 1.7 million U.S. adults, and the prevalence of the disease—largely preventable—continues to rise. Like saving money for retirement, if you fail to address your health when you're still relatively young, it will come back to bite you in your later years. You'll be having more doctor visits to deal with your high blood pressure. Or you'll be scheduling regular trips to your physical therapist to combat the joint pain you struggle with from lugging around excess weight. All because you couldn't find the time.

NO ONE EVER DROWNED IN SWEAT

I've come across many people struggling to achieve their fitness goals who complain to me: "I work out all the time but don't seem to be getting anywhere." The reason is almost always the same—what they think is a workout isn't really working out. They use the foam roller and stretch for 20 minutes before getting near a weight. Then they'll do some sets of biceps curls and machine chest presses, always taking lengthy breaks to check their e-mail or send texts. There's rarely a moment when they feel stressed by the resistance they're encountering, or even slightly uncomfortable. The only way they sweat is if the air-conditioning in the gym is broken. My point is this: simply walking through the doors of a gym does not mean you worked out.

Although I never had the chance to play with him, I got to meet and get to know Packer legend Reggie White—a Hall of Fame defensive end known as the Minister of Defense. Reggie was blessed with tremendous size and strength, but what made him special was his work ethic. He taught me that how you practice is how you're going to play. You don't take days off. You don't take plays off. Give it everything you have, all the time. Every rep counts. He told me that I could be a superstar one day. I just had to keep working every single day.

I promise the structure of the workouts in this book won't allow you to idle away your time in the gym refreshing your Twitter feed. You're basically going to be moving from the moment you start the session until the last rep. But you still need to bring maximum effort. The workouts are no longer than 45 minutes, so you have to make the most of them. Leave your work calls, family drama, and every other trouble at the door, and commit your entire self to owning that workout.

The great thing about effort is it requires no talent. You don't have to be tall, strong, fast, or athletic. Everyone has the ability to put forth their best. What separates those who are fit and healthy from those wondering why they can't be is having the mind-set and willingness to consistently commit to their workouts and nutrition plan. To endure their muscles and lungs burning from exertion, but somehow push through for one more rep. To order fruit with their sandwich instead of chips. To try to be better today than they were yesterday.

I'm not going to lie to you: getting healthy isn't always going to be pretty. But I would rather be covered in sweat at the gym than covered in clothes at the beach. When you're challenging yourself you have to learn to "love" the uncomfortable. That may mean moving more weights than you've ever attempted before, or embracing the accompanying soreness that comes with the exercise. It could be the hunger pangs you're enduring because you're monitoring your caloric intake for the first time in your life. Success isn't free. You have to work for it. But it's worth the effort. And once you start seeing the results of your sacrifice—you look better, you perform better, you feel better—the process not only becomes easier, it becomes addictive.

ROUTINE IS NOT BORING

The surest, most effective way to make regular exercise and healthy eating a part of your life is by building routines into your schedule. Much like effort, it takes no talent to develop positive routines and habits. You just need to be disciplined and consistent. If you approach the week with the notion that you'll figure out a way to fit in some workouts without planning for them, you're setting yourself up for failure. It's not a regimen that will work long-term. Just as you would for meetings or appointments at work, you need to actively arrange blocks of time when you can hit the gym. This will help you form positive, sustainable habits. As Olympian Jim Ryun said: "Motivation is what gets you started. Habit is what keeps you going."

Same goes for your nutrition. If you don't regularly shop in the produce aisle and take the time to prepare healthy meals—expecting to somehow find one during your lunch hour when presented with an array of tempting gut-busting alternatives—you're not being realistic. This book contains numerous, simple recipes that take little time to cook up, pack a nutritional punch, and taste great. Even if the extent of your cooking skills is making restaurant reservations, you can still figure a way to eat smart.

But before we get to that, it's time to hit the gym. Prepare to be uncomfortable, and love every minute of it.

DETER

TO G

MINED
T FIT

WORKOUT PROGRAMS OVERVIEW

You'll have to do what others won't, to achieve what others don't.

—Les Brown

I'll admit it: I love working out. Call me crazy, but I get excited anytime I get to push, pull, and perspire. After all, sweat is nothing more than making fat cry. But I also know I enjoy it because after so many years of doing it professionally and recreationally, I've discovered the most effective and efficient ways to train. I've seen the results firsthand on myself and the numerous people I've worked with at my gym. If you only want to lose weight, cutting back on calories and following my meal plans will suffice. If you want to be truly fit and experience optimum health, you need to work out. You need to be dogged in your training to achieve the highest level of fitness in your life. I'm going to show you the best way I know how.

The workout regimens in this book are a combination of both full-body and body-part sessions designed to build lean muscle mass, improve cardiovascular health, and increase overall athleticism. There are three workout templates: the basic and intermediate programs will focus on fat loss, muscle growth, and endurance; the advanced program will add elements of strength and power production. Equipment and exercise options make the programs versatile enough to be performed at a standard, home, or "cross-style" gym.

What's unique about these workouts is that instead of more traditional bodybuilding training paradigms that focus on exact numbers of reps and sets of exercises to be completed in a particular workout, these circuit-style workouts are structured to increase work capacity over a specific time period. For instance, most people are familiar with the tried-and-true 3×10 setup: you do a set of 10 repetitions of a certain movement, rest, and then repeat it two more times for a total of 30 reps. Nice and simple and all told it may take about five minutes to perform. But what if in that same five minutes you managed to perform more than double the number of reps by limiting rest and using more muscle groups, for a greater metabolic expenditure. And the next time you performed the workout you managed to execute even more reps in the same amount of time, or the identical number but with greater resistance. Either way, your body will be adapting to an increased amount of load, which promotes change.

In my programs, instead of focusing on a confined rep range, you will gauge and improve your weekly performance by increasing your overall output in terms of either more work or increased weight in the same amount of time. This type of anaerobic training combines both strength and cardio benefits, improving body composition, increasing postworkout metabolic rate (the afterburn effect), and eliciting greater cardiovascular endurance and VO_2 max (the amount of oxygen your body can use during exercise). A person's overall fitness is essentially measured by his or her ability to do a physical task—lift a certain amount of weight, run a set distance—and the time it takes to do it. An athlete who can complete 100 push-ups in 3 minutes is fitter than an athlete who takes twice as long; a runner who completes a mile in under 6 minutes is in better condition than one who needs more than 7. If you're consistently doing more work in less time, you're increasing your fitness level and reaping all the health benefits that come along with it. By being pushed to your own work capacity you're building greater horsepower for your body's motor.

SOUND TOO DIFFICULT?

Not if you know which exercises to perform and the proper sequence in which to perform them. Plus, this type of challenge-based training is more fun and focused than the typical gym workout. Since you're working against yourself with a specific goal, you'll be motivated to stay committed and intense each session. Distractions like the talking heads on the TV in the gym or the junk e-mail on your phone will pale in comparison to cranking out a few more quality reps. That's how you'll get in the best shape of your life. And trust me, if stripping your body of fat and replacing it with lean muscle is what you're after, there's no better way. Studies have consistently shown that this type of training is clearly more effective at elevating a person's resting metabolic rate and postexercise oxygen consumption than steady-state aerobic activity (spinning your wheels on a treadmill).

You'll start out by determining which of the three workout plans is appropriate for you. If you were listening to a Walkman the last time you hit the gym, there's no shame in starting out with the beginner program. Believe me, you will still be challenged. Plus, it's always better to start slow and gain confidence with each successful workout. If you're well conditioned, having been training for several years, then you can jump right to the intermediate level. Still, I recommend starting at the lower rep ranges to see how your body handles this type of training. And unless you're an absolute beast in the weight room, I strongly urge you not to try the advanced level before proving yourself at every stage of the intermediate level. Once you see the workouts, you'll understand why—I do them with the top trainers and strongest athletes at my gym, and we often struggle to complete them. But before we get into the details of each program, I want to explain a few training concepts first.

WARM-UP

Like any sports car, you don't want to rev your engine at high speeds before getting it warmed up. Working out cold can lead to poor performance and potential injury. However, while warming up is obviously important, I'm not a huge fan of people who turn their preworkout routine into a lengthy soft-tissue massage and stretching session. I also think it's overkill to perform multiple sets of mobility exercises and dynamic movements for each muscle group. Everybody is different, and some people may need a little more warming up than others, but a warm-up still shouldn't take as long as the workout.

And keeping it short doesn't mean it won't be effective. If you've got some tight spots—lower back, hamstrings—you can start with foam rolling to loosen those areas. Then you can transition to some light activity to get the blood pumping. That could be an easy run on the treadmill, a quick bike ride, a few minutes of jump rope, jumping jacks, or light kettlebell swings. Follow that with dynamic stretches such as alternating lunges with rotation reaches, hand walkouts, arm circles, shoulder rolls, and the list goes on. Spend the most time on body parts that take the longest to warm up. Then finish up with movement preparation. Do short sets with light weights of the exercises you'll be executing for that workout. The whole warm-up should take no more than 10 minutes.

Get loose, get a little lathered up, and get to work.

REST AS NEEDED

The workouts are set up as circuits consisting of four to seven exercises that draw on different muscle groups and energy systems. The movements are meant to be done back-to-back and when you've completed the circuit, you repeat the grouping until you hit ten rounds or 45 minutes of training—whichever comes first.

SO WHEN DO YOU REST?

That's up to you. While many training systems program rest into the workouts, I'm not a big proponent of it. Under certain circumstances, such as training purely to increase strength in a particular movement—such as the bench press, deadlift, or squat—I appreciate the value of taking extended time between sets. In our advanced workouts that deal primarily with strength and power, fewer reps and exercises are performed each round. So with less volume and heavier weights, there's greater opportunity to rest and recover.

But if your goal is to strip fat and build lean muscle, then I find you're better off setting your own pace. If you breeze through a set of squats, I don't see the value of taking a minute break when the time it takes to transition to the next exercise will easily suffice as your rest. On the other hand, if you're on your seventh round of the workout, and a set of walking dumbbell lunges turns your legs to quivering jelly—I love that feeling—you may need to gather yourself for a bit longer before taking on the next movement.

It's definitely a sophisticated way to train, especially for beginners. But I strongly endorse it because:

1. It lets you set your own limitations—Every person's physiology and recovery skills are different. Resting as needed allows you to better understand your body, what you're capable of, and where you need to draw the line.

2. If done right, you work your tail off—I don't think getting enough rest between sets is the problem for most people. In fact, it's usually the opposite. People don't work hard enough in the gym. They're concerned much more with cranking out texts than with their next set. The way my workouts are structured, you've got to be focused and efficient or you won't complete them. You've got to push yourself to be better than you were the time before. Sore? Tired? Out of breath? Sweaty? Good . . . it's working.

NEVER SACRIFICE FORM FOR TIME

One of the natural pitfalls of trying to beat a running clock is sloppy form. You're so eager to improve on your previous time for a particular workout that you compromise technique. Bad idea. This becomes even more prevalent as you begin to tire. Besides cheating yourself of the full value of the movement, more important is the greater likelihood of sustaining an injury. As legendary UCLA men's basketball coach John Wooden said: "Be quick, but don't hurry."

As much as I want you to exert maximum effort, I also want you to use good judgment. Lift and lower the weights in a safe, controlled fashion. The eccentric phase of a movement—the lowering portion—has been shown to promote the greatest muscle growth. Not working at all against that resistance by dropping the weight as quickly as possible is not taking full advantage of the exercise. Plus, you don't want to be the guy at the gym who's mocked for bouncing his weights on the floor.

Along those lines, when you start to notice your form breaking down and your muscles failing, take more rest. Pacing yourself during these workouts is not only critical for finishing them, it's essential to preserving your long-term ability to perform. The purpose of training is to stimulate the body, not annihilate it. You should feel tested by the workout, even a little spent, but not to the point of complete exhaustion. If being horizontal is the only position you can hold after a workout, you know you crossed the line into bodily abuse.

DON'T HANG YOUR HEAD IF YOU DON'T FINISH

Not every challenge can be met. My teams didn't win every football game we played, nor did I always put up great individual numbers. Sometimes the day beats you. And that's okay. We have to face these types of adversities in order to know what we must do to improve. The workouts in this book are no different. Even though I've designed them to be scaled to any ability level, they're going to test your resolve. And sometimes, depending on the exercises, weights, and reps you choose, the workout will win. You're not going to be able to finish. Again, that's okay. In fact, that's exactly what I want. I want this to be a growth process where you keep striving for what you once thought impossible.

And I'm going to let you in on a little secret: I often don't finish the workouts. I'll try one of the advanced workouts and get too ambitious in terms of weight used or rep total, and either fatigue or the clock will be my undoing. If you're in the middle of a workout, grinding through dumbbell chest presses with pulsing pecs and shaky arms, failing on your 6th rep of 10, then call it a day. Be proud you took on a formidable challenge and gave it everything you had. You may not be there yet, but you're closer than you were yesterday. Just don't be satisfied. Whatever your score, beat it the next time. And the time after that.

I've been working out most of my life. At least, I thought I was working out. Prior to training with Donald, I was a member of the YMCA taking group classes and doing my own workouts. I stayed in relatively good shape and as I approached forty, I felt I had reached my fitness peak and had basically plateaued. However, when I turned forty, I joined Donald's gym and that's when working out took on a whole new meaning for me.

Donald's style of training is high intensity, high energy. Extremely high from start to finish. Because of his background as a world-class professional athlete, he knows what the human body is capable of and he expects more out of his clients than the average certified trainer. He introduced me to high-intensity resistance training, which I had stayed away from for fear of "bulking up." But just as Donald told me on day one, "his way" will get me in the best shape of my life, no matter what my age.

Donald comes up with fun and innovative classes that push you right up to your limits, without ever asking more of you than you can handle. If you don't give your full effort, Donald knows and he'll call you on it every time. There's just something special about a guy who makes you do things you don't want to do, or even thought you were capable of. I'm no professional athlete, I'm a mom of two. Some days you just don't feel like doing burpees, but Donald will drop down on the floor with you and help you push through it.

The greatest testament to his training is that I can honestly say I'm in better shape at forty-four than I was at twenty-four. I can really see a difference in my body and fitness level since joining Donald's gym. My legs are stronger with more definition and I've sculpted the strong shoulders and arms that I've always wanted. Best of all, I feel great and look forward to his workouts. Although they may be tough, his positive energy and enthusiasm are contagious and help his entire class be the best version of themselves.

Jackie Burleson
Coppell, Texas

CHAPTER 3

EXERCISE GARAGE

*It is a shame to grow old without seeing the beauty
and strength of which your body is capable.*

—Socrates

Perhaps the only thing worse than not working out is working out with improper form. The purpose of training is improvement, not injury. So before we jump into the workouts, which are built from the exercises in this chapter, I recommend that you first spend some time reviewing these movements and internalizing the proper form. A barbell back squat is a wonderfully effective total body movement, but if performed incorrectly one bad rep can wreck a knee or lower back, not to mention staple you to the floor. This chapter provides step-by-step, photographic demonstrations of proper technique for all the exercises in the workout programs. These are the tools that will turn your body into a fierce, racing machine. However, this is just a healthy smattering of what you can do. An endless supply of exercises and variations can be plugged into these workouts. Expand your toolbox—be creative and resourceful and seek out the possibilities. But no matter what exercises you do choose, always strive to employ the best technique possible.

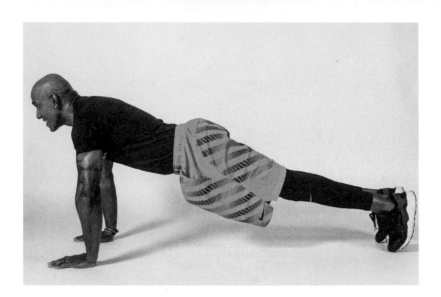

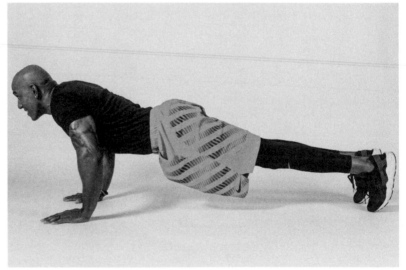

UPPER BODY PUSH

PUSH-UPS

This staple needs little introduction. Start in a plank position with your hands just outside shoulder width apart, back flat, core tight, and toes pressing into the floor. Lower your chest to just above the floor, not allowing your elbows to flare out excessively; then drive up until your arms are completely straight. Keep your body in a tight, straight line—no hip hinge or sagging butt.

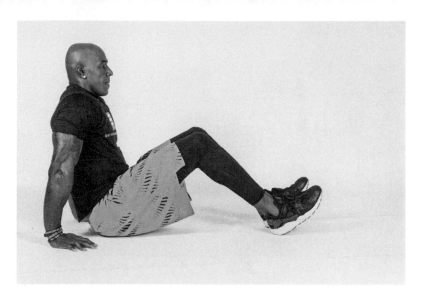

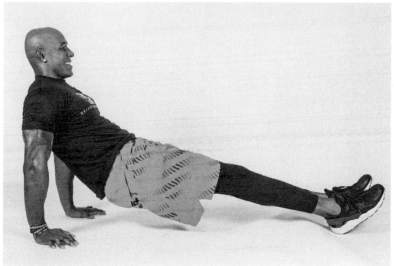

FLOOR DIPS

Sit with your knees bent and your heels digging into the floor. Place your hands just behind your backside with your fingers pointed toward your feet and elbows pointed away from you. Drive your feet and hands into the floor to bring your hips off the ground into a reverse tabletop position. Slowly bend your elbows while trying to keep your body in a straight line. When your backside gets just above the floor, straighten your arms to return to the starting reverse tabletop position. If you want to add in a cardio component, add in walking on your hands and feet like a crab.

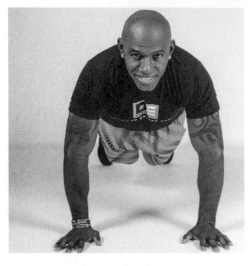

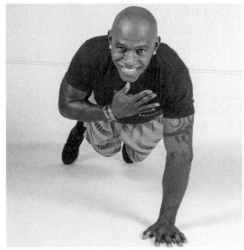

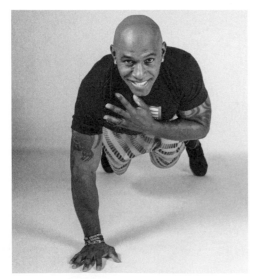

SHOULDER TAPS

Get into a plank position with your hands just outside shoulder width, core braced, back flat, and toes pushing through the floor. Maintaining this posture and not allowing your body to sway, lift your right hand off the floor and touch your left shoulder. Return it to the floor and repeat the movement with your left hand touching your right shoulder. While this tests shoulder stability, increasing the speed will elevate the core component. Or add a push-up between taps to add a strength element and increase the difficulty level.

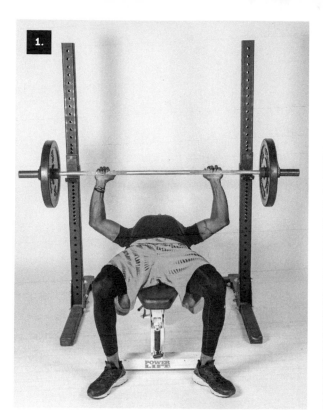

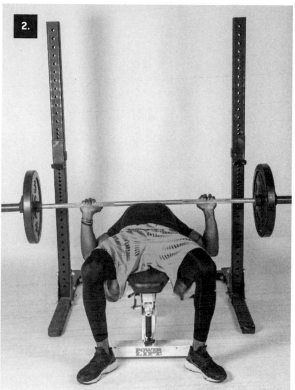

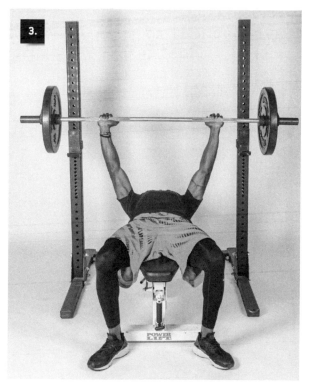

BENCH PRESS

Everyone's favorite measuring stick. Lie on a flat bench with your eyes directly underneath the bar. Grab the bar with a grip slightly outside shoulder width—a good cue for proper placement is to make sure your forearms are perpendicular to the floor. Keep your hips firmly placed against the bench with a slight arch in the lower back and your shoulder blades packed by squeezing them down and together. Put your feet flat on the floor and establish tension from your toes up to your hands. Unrack the bar, making sure to keep your shoulder blades packed. Lower the bar to the center of your chest just below the nipples, keeping your elbows tight to the body at a 45-degree angle. Drive the bar up and slightly backward until arms are fully extended.

VARIATION: INCLINE BENCH PRESS

Lie on an adjustable bench with the back set at a 30- to 45-degree angle. This will increase emphasis on the upper part of your chest muscles. As the angle increases, the amount of weight you're capable of using will decrease. Follow the same technique as the bench press, except that when you lower the bar it should touch higher up on the chest, just below the clavicle.

A NOTE ON GRIP

Grab the bar with an overhand grip slightly outside shoulder width, with your thumbs around the bar. Make sure your forearms are perpendicular to the floor. Advanced lifters sometimes employ a thumbless grip (shown above), positioning the bar lower in the hand and more directly over the forearm; this can generate more power, but since the bar can roll off and cause injury, this grip is not advised for beginners. If you are attempting the thumbless grip, do it only with a spotter or in a power rack equipped with safety pins.

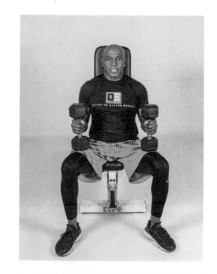

SEATED DUMBBELL
SHOULDER PRESS

Grab a pair of dumbbells and sit on a military or utility bench with upright back support. Place the end of the dumbbell on each knee and raise your legs one at a time to help lift the dumbbells to around ear level. At this point make sure your palms are facing forward. Keeping your abdominals tight, feet firmly planted into the floor, and upper back flat against the bench, extend your arms to press the weights over your head so they nearly touch. After a brief pause, slowly lower the weights back to ear level and repeat for the allotted reps. For a bigger ask on the core, the press can also be performed while standing with the feet about shoulder width apart.

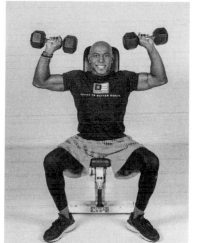

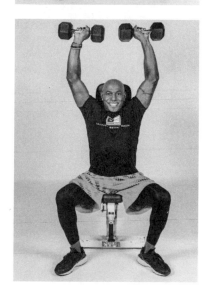

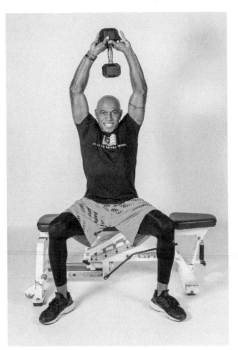
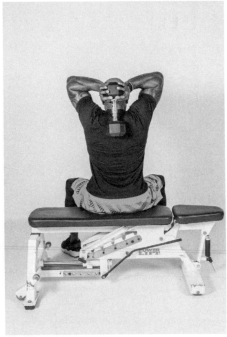

SEATED OVERHEAD TRICEPS EXTENSION

Sit on a sturdy box or bench with your feet just outside shoulder width apart. Grab one side of a dumbbell with both hands and lift it overhead until both arms are extended. The weight should rest in the palms of your hands, which face the ceiling. Lower the weight behind your head by bending at the elbows as your upper arms remain beside your ears and nearly perpendicular to the floor. Allow your forearms to go slightly past parallel to the floor before using your triceps to press the weight back to the starting position. Be sure to control the weight through the movement so it doesn't bonk you on the back of the head. This exercise can also be performed while standing.

FLOOR EXTENSION/SUPERMAN

Lie facedown on the floor on your belly. Extend your legs out straight behind you with your arms by your sides, or crossed on the floor under your chin with your hands stacked. Slowly raise your chest and lower legs off the floor. Be careful not to arch your back too severely. Pause briefly before slowly returning to the starting position. To make this move more challenging, extend your arms in front of you and raise them along with your legs. It will look like you're flying and that's why the exercise is commonly called a Superman.

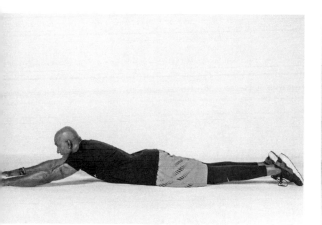

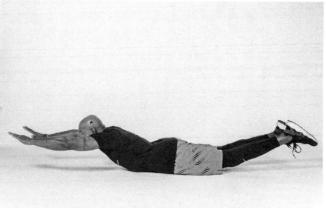

PULL-UP

There's arguably no exercise better at building the upper back. Grab an elevated fixed bar using a pronated grip (hands facing away from you) with your hands slightly wider than shoulder width. Start with your arms fully extended and your feet raised off the floor. Initiate the movement by driving your elbows toward the floor and squeezing your shoulder blades together. Continue to raise your body until your chin is just above the bar. To complete the exercise, slowly lower your body until your arms are fully extended (dead hang). This move can also be done with a supinated grip (hands facing you) with your hands positioned just inside shoulder width on the bar. Otherwise known as a chin-up, it involves the biceps more and is generally easier to perform than a pull-up. Once you get proficient at this movement, you can wear a weight belt or hold a dumbbell between your feet for extra resistance and major back gains.

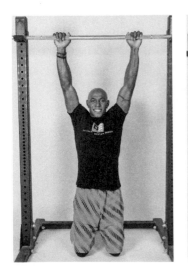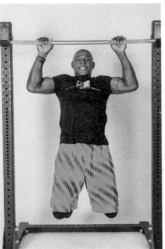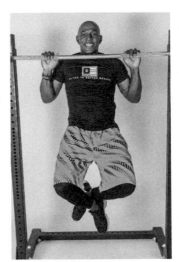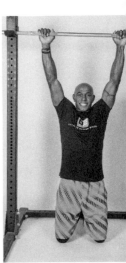

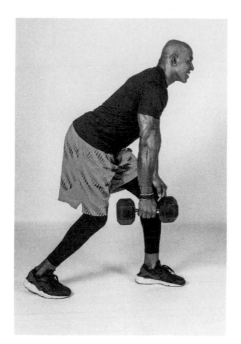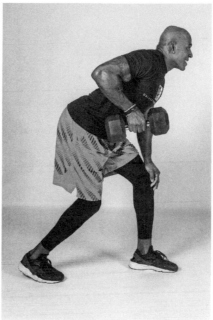

BENT-OVER ONE-ARM DUMBBELL ROW

Holding a dumbbell in your dominant hand with a neutral grip, assume a staggered stance with your opposite foot forward. Bend at your hips to lower your torso so that it's nearly parallel to the floor and place your nondominant hand on your forward knee. Alternatively, you can put your hand on a box, a bench, or any steady object for support. Let the dumbbell hang at arm's length from your shoulder. While keeping your upper body tight—don't round your back—and your posture steady, pull the dumbbell up to your ribs and squeeze your shoulder blade toward your spine. Pause briefly and control the weight back down to the hanging position. Repeat for the allotted reps; then alternate working arm and stance.

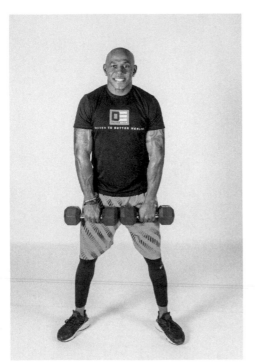
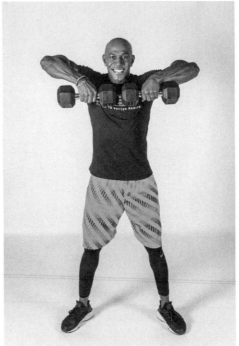

UPRIGHT ROW

Stand holding a dumbbell in each hand with an overhand grip, just inside shoulder width. Your arms should be extended with a slight bend in the elbows as the weight rests against your thighs. Engaging your shoulders, raise your elbows up and to the sides as you lift the weights—try to keep them close to the body—to just underneath your chin. Pause briefly and lower the weights under control. Keep your elbows above your forearms during the movement and maintain a rigid torso; don't rock back when lifting the dumbbells, or fall forward when lowering them. This exercise can also be done with a barbell, which allows for heavier weights to be lifted, but can be difficult for people with wrist issues.

FRONT RAISE

Stand holding a dumbbell in each hand at arm's length, positioned at thigh level with an overhand grip. While maintaining a rigid upper body and a slight bend in the elbow, lift one of the dumbbells up until it is just about even with the shoulder. Pause briefly; then lower under control. Make sure not to rock back on the ascent, or to lean forward when lowering. Repeat with the other arm. This movement can also be done with both dumbbells moving simultaneously.

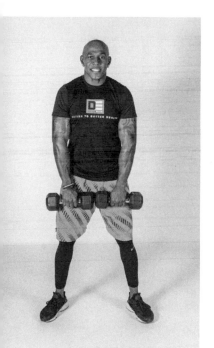
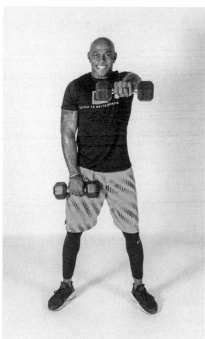
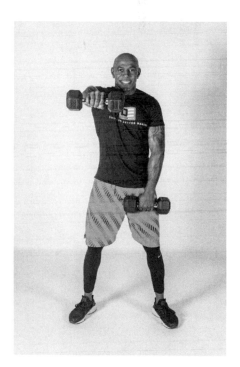

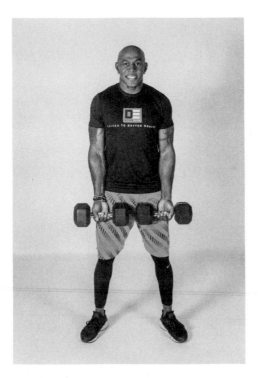

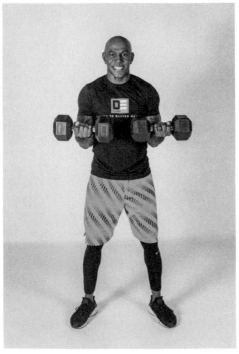

DUMBBELL CURL

This is the classic shirtsleeve expander. Stand with your feet about shoulder width apart while holding a dumbbell in each hand with your palms facing forward. Maintaining a rigid torso—no rocking or leaning back—and elbows tucked by your sides, curl both dumbbells up toward your head. Your upper arms should not be moving, only your forearms. Raise the weights until they're at shoulder height and the biceps are fully contracted. Hold the squeeze briefly before lowering the weights back down to the starting position. You can vary the movement by alternating one arm at a time and/or by starting with the palms facing down (reverse curl) or each other (hammer curl).

SQUAT

Stand with your feet shoulder width apart, or slightly wider. Point your toes straight ahead or a bit flared out. Lower yourself into a squat by pushing your hips back as if sitting in a chair. Allow your knees to track out toward your toes while keeping your back flat. Go down until your upper thighs are parallel to the floor, or just past parallel. Your arms can remain at your sides or out in front of you. Drive upward by pushing through the middle of your feet.

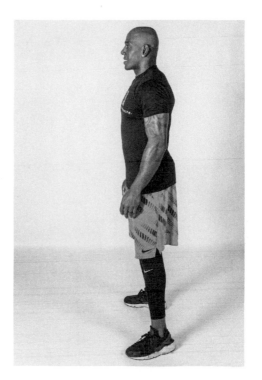

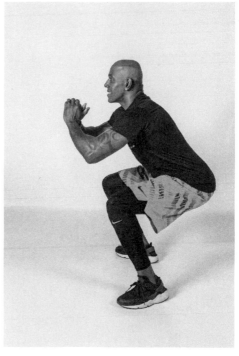

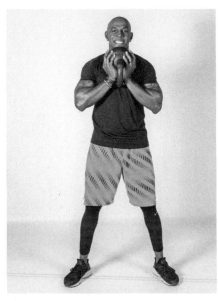

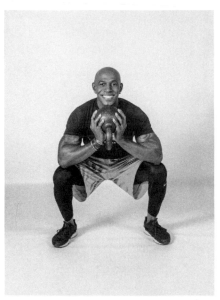

GOBLET SQUAT

This is a safe and effective method for adding resistance to the squat, as well as ingraining proper movement pattern. Hold a kettlebell by the horns or base (bottom up), or one end of a dumbbell, by your chest. With your feet just outside shoulder width and feet pointed out slightly, sit down between your knees. Drop to a depth low enough so that your elbows touch the insides of your knees. Be sure to keep your chest up to prevent any rounding of the back or a forward lean. Stand back up, returning to the starting position, and repeat.

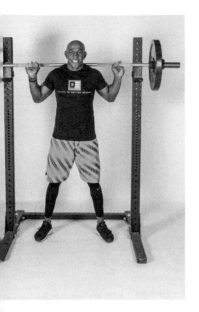 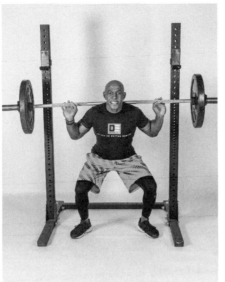 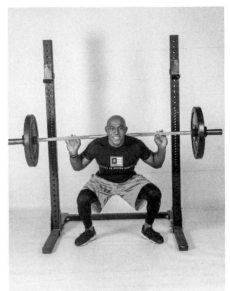

BACK SQUAT

Place a bar behind your neck and rest it across your upper trapezius muscles. Pulling your shoulder blades down and together will create a nice "shelf" for the bar to sit on. You don't want it contacting your neck. Grab the bar with a wide, overhand grip and squeeze tightly. Keep your chest high and maintain a rigid core as you descend into a squat. Remember to keep a flat back—if it begins to round during the movement, the weight is probably too heavy—and your knees are behind your toes. Once your upper thighs are at least parallel to the floor, push through your feet to power the weight back up to the starting position. Add these regularly to your workouts and you'll see noticeable improvements to the size and shape of your legs, and why so many call this the "King of All Exercises."

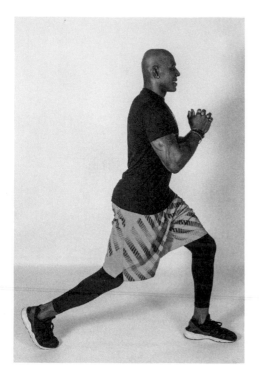

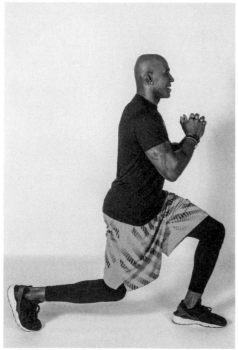

LUNGE

Standing with your feet about shoulder width apart, with one foot take a big step forward, landing heel first. The front foot should be flat on the floor, while the back foot is up on the toes. Your upper body should be relatively upright. Descend by bending the front knee until the back knee almost touches the floor. Your front knee should be at just about a 90-degree angle, and should not go past the toes. Push through the front foot and raise your hips to bring the lead leg back to the starting position. You can complete all reps one leg at a time, or by alternating.

STEP-UPS

Stand facing a box, bench, or raised platform with your feet shoulder width apart.
Step your nondominant foot (that's my left)
up on top of the object so that the entire
foot is flat. Push through the left foot to
lift your body up. Make sure to extend up
using only the working leg—the right leg
is along for the ride. When your left leg is
straight, you can gently place your right
foot on the object. Pause briefly; then
step off with your right leg. As soon as it
contacts the floor, step up with your left leg
again. Complete all your reps with one leg
before switching to the other.

NOTE

It's often a good idea to start unilateral
exercises with your nondominant (weaker)
limb when you're fresher. Following with
your stronger/dominant side ensures you'll
be more likely to maintain good form when
fatiguing.

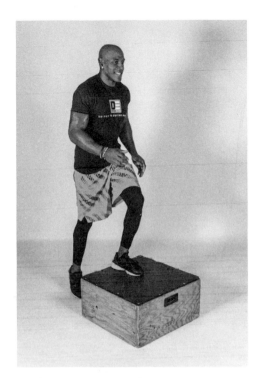

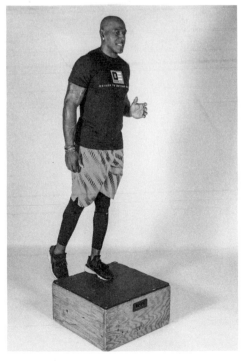

DEADLIFT

If the squat is the king of all exercises, here's your queen. Nothing screams power like lifting a massive weight off the floor. 1) Stand with feet shoulder width apart with a loaded bar just above the middle of your feet. Push your hips back until your hands are around knee level or you feel a stretch in your hamstrings. Then bend your knees until your hands can grasp the bar in an overhand grip with straight arms just outside your legs. Roll the bar back slightly until it is directly underneath your shoulders, which should be just in front of or grazing your shins. Your lower back should be slightly arched—no rounding. Grip the bar tightly and tense up your body from head to toe. 2) Push through the floor to straighten your legs and initiate the lift from the floor. Your lower back should maintain its arch, with the bar staying close to your body. This is critical. Put too much stress on your lower back and you won't be able to tie your shoes for a week. 3) Once the bar passes the knees, bring your hips forward and squeeze your shoulder blades together, opening up your chest. You should be standing tall with your shoulders back and the bar at arm's length against your body. 4) Return the weight to the floor under control by reversing the motion, keeping the bar in contact with your body. Since the bar tends to drag against your shins, it's not uncommon to wear athletic pants when deadlifting.

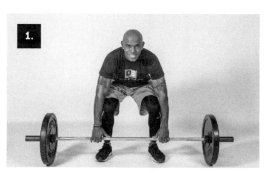

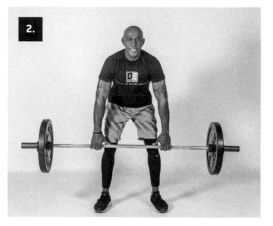

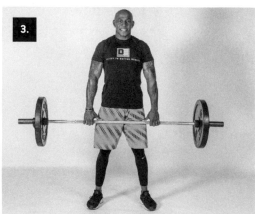

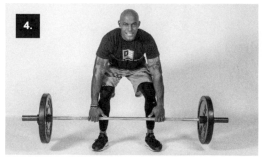

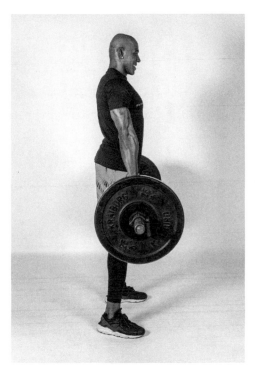
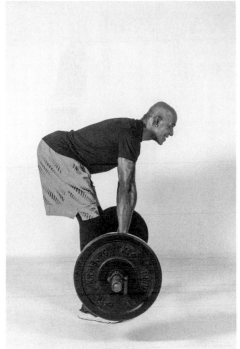

ROMANIAN DEADLIFT

Also commonly called a stiff-legged deadlift, this exercise starts in the finishing position of a conventional deadlift: feet shoulder width apart, torso straight, shoulders back, bar in an overhand grip at arm's length resting against your upper thighs. To initiate the movement, push your hips back to lower the bar until it's just below your knees to mid-shin level and you feel a stretch in your hamstrings. Your knees may bend some, but it should not be excessive. The bar should stay close to your body, and your back should maintain its natural arch throughout. To complete the lifting phase, bring your hips forward and stick your chest out, pulling the bar along your thighs to raise it to the starting position. You should feel the stretch in your glutes/hamstrings rather than powering the bar with your lower back.

BURPEE

Nobody likes these, so you know they're effective. With your feet about shoulder width apart, squat down and place your hands on the floor just in front of and outside your feet. Jump both feet back so that you're in a plank position. From there, lower your body to the floor to perform a push-up, returning to the plank position. Then jump your feet forward to just inside and below your hands. Explode up into the air, essentially performing a squat jump, reaching your arms straight up. Land softly with bent knees and repeat for the required reps. Make sure you've got a towel handy.

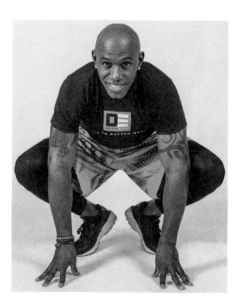
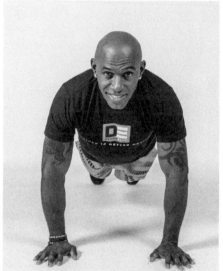
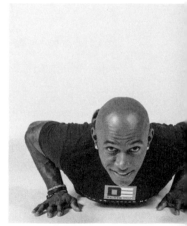

DONKEY KICKS

Get on all fours with your hands under your shoulders and your knees below your hips. Bracing your core, lift one leg off the floor toward the ceiling so that it forms a straight line with your upper body, and the bottom of your foot is facing the ceiling. Return the leg to the starting position and repeat with the other leg. To perform a more advanced version, lean your weight forward onto your hands, rise up off your knees, and simultaneously kick both legs up and back. After fully extending your legs, pull your knees quickly toward your chest so your feet can "catch" your legs before they hit the floor. Do these explosively and they'll really kick your butt.

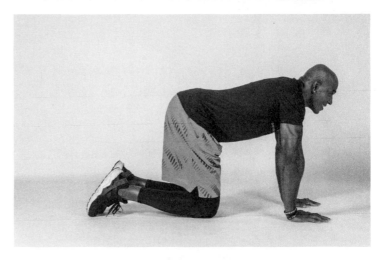

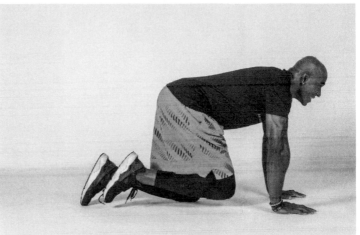

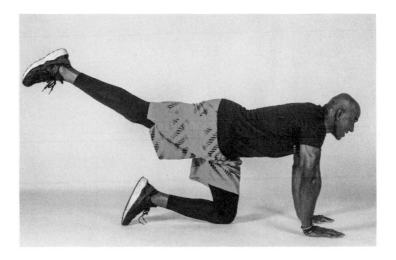

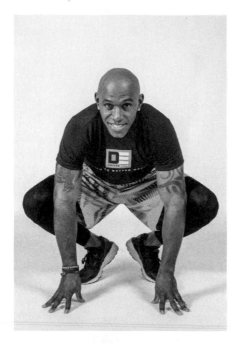

FROG THRUST

Stand with your feet outside shoulder width. Sink your hips down and bend your knees so that you're in a deep squat with your backside just off the ground. Place your hands just inside your feet. At this point you should look like a frog. In one continuous motion, explode up, straightening your knees and hips and raising your hands over your head. You can either jump as high as possible or jump for distance. Land softly with bent knees and immediately drop back down into the starting (frog) position to repeat the movement. You'll need a good amount of space and a good set of lungs to perform this one.

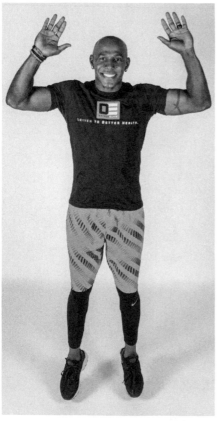

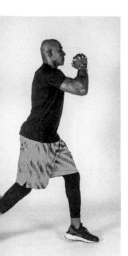 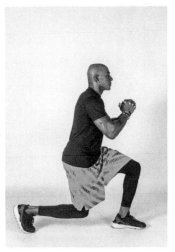 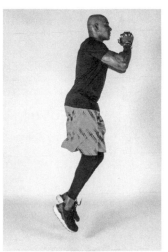 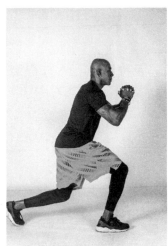

SPLIT SQUAT JUMPS

Take a staggered stance with one foot out in front of the body, and the other foot placed behind. Maintain an upright posture as you dip the body down, bending both knees. Keep your front foot planted firmly on the floor, while the heel on the back foot is slightly raised. When the back knee is just above the floor, jump upward as forcefully as possible, repositioning the legs in the opposite positions upon landing. Immediately repeat the movement, continuing to switch legs in the air with each repetition. Do enough of these in a row and your legs will feel like Jell-O.

THRUSTER

This move is a hybrid/combo of a front squat and a shoulder push press. With your feet in an athletic stance, hold a barbell or pair of dumbbells at shoulder height. While maintaining a strong core, drop down into a squat position, keeping the weights at the original rack position. Explode out of the down position, using your legs, hips, and upward momentum to help your shoulders and arms propel the bar or dumbbells overhead. Bring the weights back down to shoulder position and immediately repeat. Use enough weight and this movement is a killer.

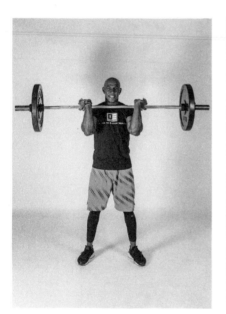 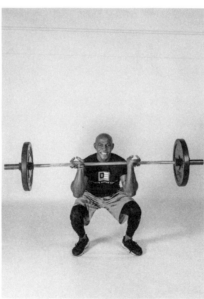 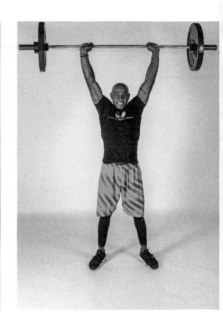

DUMBBELL UP-DOWN

Stand with your feet shoulder width apart, arms at your sides holding a dumbbell in each hand. Keeping a flat back and braced core, bend your knees and lower the dumbbells to the floor just outside your feet. While holding the dumbbells and pressing them into the floor, kick your feet back, landing in a plank position. Immediately push through your toes, jumping your feet back underneath your shoulders so that you're in a low squat. Stand up holding the dumbbells to return to the starting position.

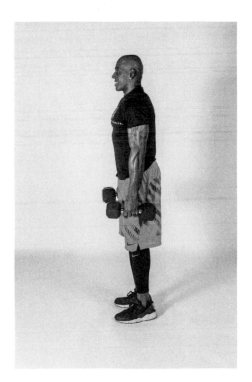

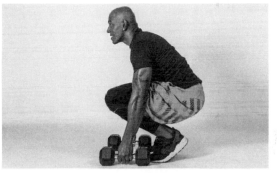

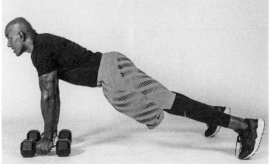

RENEGADE ROW

Place two kettlebells or hexagonal dumbbells (if available) on the floor about shoulder width apart. Holding the weights, get into a plank position, up on your toes with your feet outside your shoulders. This wider base will help with balance. Bracing your core—try to keep the hips parallel throughout—and pushing one weight into the floor, row the other weight to your chest. Pause briefly and return the weight to the floor. Repeat on the other side. This also doubles as a great core exercise.

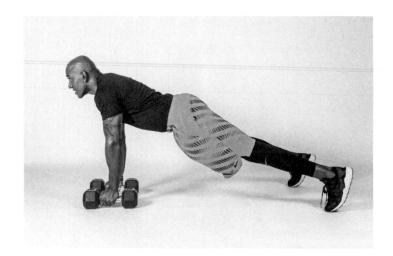

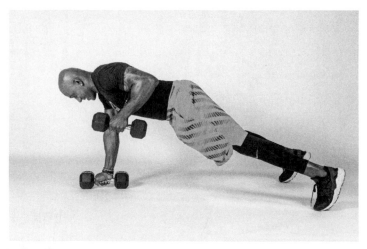

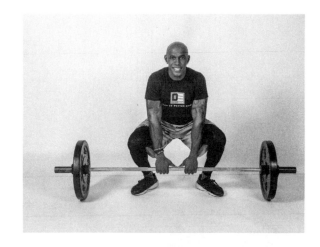

SUMO DEADLIFT HIGH PULL

With the bar on the floor, take a wide stance with your feet slightly pointed out. Sit your hips back and bend your knees so your arms lower to grasp the bar inside your knees with an overhand grip, all the while maintaining a flat back. Push your feet into the floor, extend your knees and hips, and power the weight off the floor. As the bar reaches midthigh, continue pulling by driving your elbows back toward the ceiling. At completion of the movement you should be up on your toes, body fully extended, having moved the bar from the shins to just underneath the chin. It's an explosive move, so be careful of the bar's finishing height—smack into your jaw and you could be minus some teeth. Return the bar to the floor before initiating the next rep.

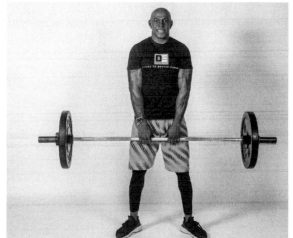

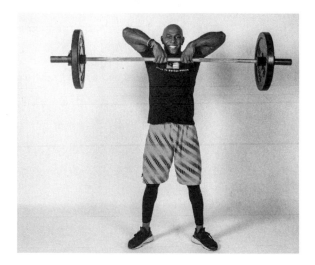

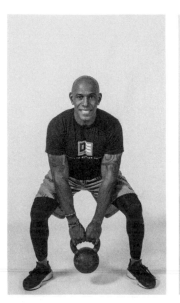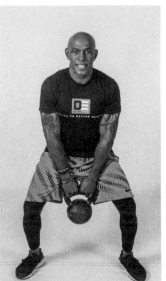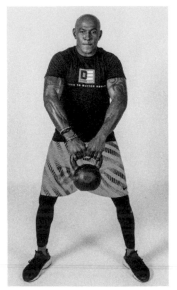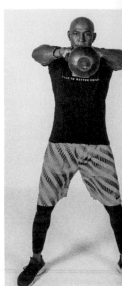

KETTLEBELL/DUMBBELL SWING

Stand with your feet about shoulder width apart. Grasp a kettlebell by its horns, or one of the ends of a dumbbell, with your palms facing you. With a flat back, braced core, and slight knee bend, allow the weight to travel back between your legs so it's just under your backside. This will bring your shoulders forward and your forearms in touch with your inner thighs, creating a hip hinge. Forcefully drive your hips forward to propel the bell into the air. Use your arms and shoulders to control the bell, but don't engage them to lift the weight. The bell should travel only as high as the hip hinge and thrust dictates, feeling almost weightless at its highest point. Control the bell on the descent, allowing it to travel back between your legs to spur another hip hinge. Guys, make sure you allow enough clearance between the bell and your valuables. Immediately execute the next rep; it's a continuous, fluid motion designed to generate speed.

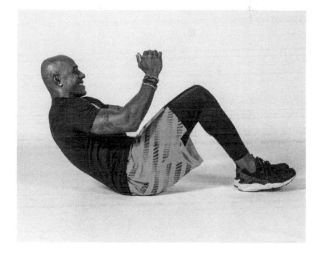

CORE

FULL SIT-UPS

Another old standby that ab-solutely works (okay, not my best). Lie down faceup, with your knees bent and your feet flat on the floor at a comfortable distance from your backside. Lace your fingers behind your head or cross your arms on your chest. Brace your abs and curl your body up to your knees. Be careful not to pull your neck forward or extend it well ahead of your spine. Lower yourself in a controlled manner, slowly placing your back on the floor one vertebra at a time.

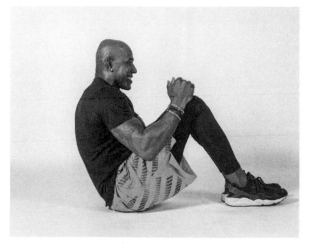

TOE TOUCHES

Lie down faceup, with your legs straight and your feet flexed so that your toes are pointing toward the ceiling. It's acceptable to have a slight bend in the knees. Extend your arms straight over your head, and lift your legs so that your body forms an *L* shape or 90-degree angle. This is your starting position. Keeping your lower back in contact with the floor, contract your abs and lift your chest toward your knees to reach your hands toward your toes. Slowly lower your torso and arms back to the starting position.

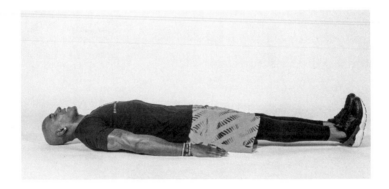

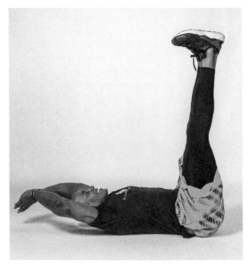
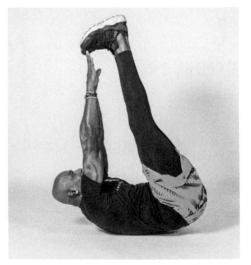

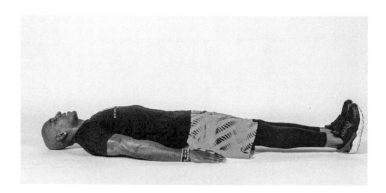

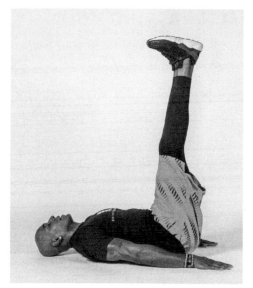
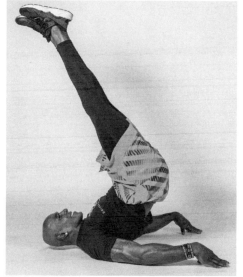

HIP LIFTS

Lie on your back with arms by your sides, palms on the floor. Extend your legs as straight as possible—a little bend is acceptable—along the floor and flex your feet so that your toes are pointing toward the ceiling. Lift your hips and backside off the floor toward the ceiling. Make sure your core is powering the movement, and you're not pressing your hands into the floor to lift your hips. As your hips curl toward your head, it's fine if your feet also drift in that direction, but not excessively. Slowly lower your hips back to the floor to complete the exercise. You can also perform this movement while lying on a bench.

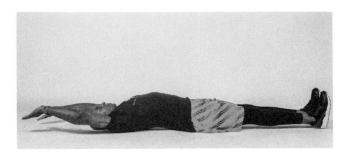

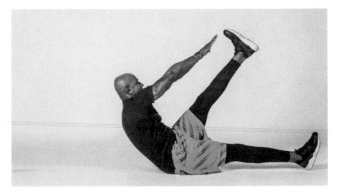

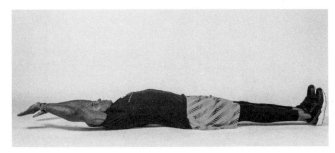

ALTERNATING V-UP

Lie flat on your back with your legs extended and touching, and arms straight overhead. Keeping your core tight and back flat, simultaneously lift your left leg and torso off the floor, reaching across your body with your right hand toward your left ankle. Lower back to the floor under control, and repeat with the opposite arm and leg. Continue in this alternating fashion until all reps are completed. Another variation is to lift both legs and arms simultaneously. And if you really want to make it difficult, hold a light medicine ball in your hands.

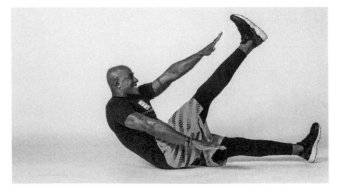

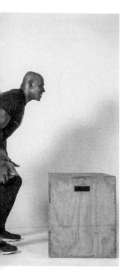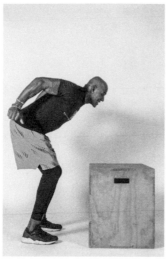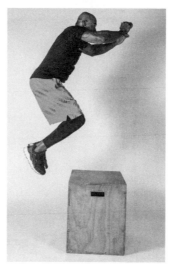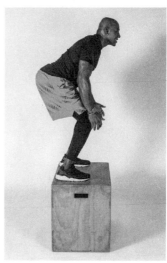

BOX JUMP

Position yourself at a comfortable jumping distance from a box or bench. Stand in an athletic position with your feet about shoulder width apart. Sink into a quarter squat—about halfway from your thighs being parallel to the floor. In one explosive motion, push your feet through the floor, extend your hips, and swing your arms to launch yourself onto the box. Relax your knees upon landing to soften the impact. Be careful not to rush these or perform them when exhausted. A missed rep could land your face on the box instead of your feet.

If you don't have access to a box or bench, or aren't yet comfortable with the exercise, you can perform a standard squat jump. Instead of leaping toward the box, go straight up in the air toward the ceiling, landing softly on the balls of your feet with bent knees. If you want to increase the difficulty, while in the air extend your arms and legs at 45-degree angles—commonly called a star jump. As you descend, quickly bring your arms and legs back toward your body, landing softly with bent knees. Another option is the broad jump. Instead of lifting your feet up to achieve maximum height, swing your legs forward in front of your body as far as possible in an attempt to jump a longer distance. Try to absorb the impact upon landing by bending at the knees and hips. A good goal to shoot for is to jump your height in distance.

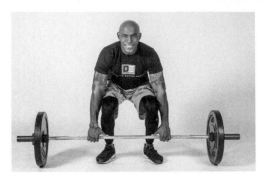

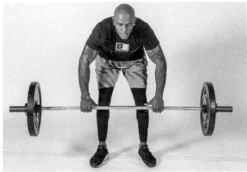

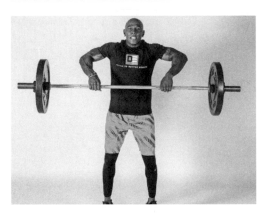

POWER CLEAN

Stand in front of a barbell with your feet hip to shoulder width apart as though you're about to jump. With an overhand grip (palms toward you), take hold of the bar slightly wider than shoulder width with your hands outside your knees and the bar right in front of your shins. Arms should be fully extended, back flat, with your hips slightly higher than your knees. To start the movement, forcefully drive your feet into the floor and extend your knees and hips to pull the bar off the ground. Keep the bar close to your body while maintaining the starting angle of your lower back (no rounding). Don't pull with your arms—keep them extended—as the move is powered by the feet/ankles, knees, and hips, commonly called triple extension. When the bar passes just above the knees, your body should be just about at full extension (on your toes). To catch the bar, bend at knees and hips and slide your feet wider to drop into a squat position, while simultaneously rotating your elbows underneath the bar until they're pointing forward. The bar should land on your shoulders with slightly open hands. A good cue is catching the bar on your shoulders just about the same time your feet hit the ground.

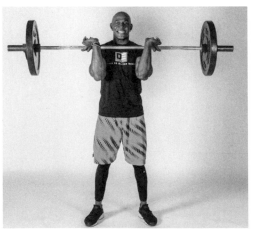

KETTLEBELL/ DUMBBELL SNATCH

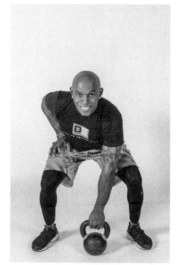
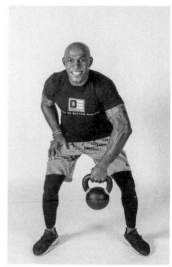

Stand with your feet about shoulder width apart with a kettlebell between them. Grasp the bell by its handle with your palm facing you. With a flat back, braced core, and slight knee bend, lift the bell and allow it to travel back between your legs so it's just under your backside. This will bring your shoulders forward and your forearm in touch with your inner thighs, creating a hip hinge. Forcefully drive your hips forward to propel the bell into the air. As it comes out from between your legs, pull up vertically with your arm close to your body, elbow leading the bell. Quickly extend and lock out your elbow to punch the bell up over your shoulder. It should be an explosive, fluid motion. Lower the bell back down to your shoulder and then let it fall between your legs before initiating the backswing to

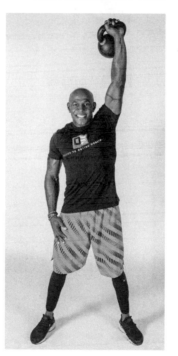
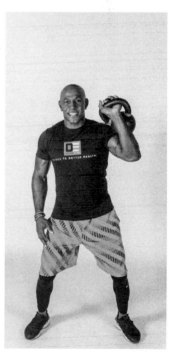

perform another rep. This movement takes a fair amount of practice to learn the finer points, so start off with a lightweight bell. If you don't have any kettlebells available, dumbbells make suitable substitutes.

CHAPTER 4

FIRST GEAR

(BEGINNER PROGRAM)

Start by doing what's necessary; then do what's possible; and suddenly you are doing the impossible. —St. Francis of Assisi

This is the jumping-off point for newbies and the out-of-practice. No matter what your experience or current conditioning level, you'll be able to modify the exercises to suit your ability. The program calls for two to three days a week of training with at least one day of rest in between. A Monday-Wednesday-Friday split would be ideal, but any combination would work as long as you're not working out on consecutive days.

At this early stage, the program is entirely composed of bodyweight exercises. If you can't manipulate your own body for an extended period of time, you're not ready for additional load. Plus, your body provides ample resistance. Ever watch top-level gymnasts? How about dancers? The professionals on *Dancing with the Stars* are muscular and ripped and it's all from moving their bodies through space. My partner, Peta Murgatroyd, was in phenomenal shape. And trust me—I had to lift her during several routines—she was solid as a rock. Dancing with her several hours a day I got down to 2 percent body fat, the lowest I have ever been. If you work intensely with your own body weight, you'll have no trouble elevating your heart rate for generalized fat loss, as well as packing on lean muscle. Don't confuse *beginner* with *easy*—you're gonna work.

As I mentioned in the Introduction, this program consists of circuit-style training.

For the beginner program it's four movements performed back-to-back with exercises in the 6- to 12-rep range. You can mix and match exercises from the Exercise Garage in Chapter 3 to come up with new circuits for variety; just make sure you follow the flow of exercise movement patterns in my sample circuits (I'll explain in greater detail shortly). And before you get started, I want you to complete an introductory test:

TEST: COMPLETE 10 ROUNDS IN 40 MIN.

		TEST WORKOUT	LEVEL 1	LEVEL 2	LEVEL 3
		EXERCISES	SETS	SETS	SETS
UPPER	1	PUSH-UPS	6	8	10
LOWER	2	SQUATS	6	8	10
CORE	3	FULL SIT-UPS	6	8	10
SPE/CARDIO	4	BURPEES	6	8	10

You will have 40 minutes to complete 10 rounds of push-ups (upper body), body-weight squats (lower body), full sit-ups (core), and burpees (speed/cardio). These are classic, great-bang-for-your-buck compound movements that will test your muscular and cardiovascular endurance. If you're completely new to training, you may want to begin with Level 1: 6 reps per movement. You may also find, no matter which level you choose, that you get through only 20 minutes of the workout before hitting a wall and can't continue. Not a problem. Everybody starts somewhere. I'll never forget my first game playing wide receiver on my high school varsity football team. I got wide open on a play and dropped what would have been a sure TD. Bounced right off my hands. I didn't look like a future pro that day. But improvement is just some hard work and belief away. Even after I became a full-time starter in the NFL, I would still ask our quarterback, Brett Favre, if the route I ran on a play was exactly what he had in mind. Always keep looking to improve.

These workouts are designed to present a challenge; so set a goal to always shoot for when you're in the gym. Next time you may get to 25 minutes and complete a few more rounds. And the time after that 30 minutes and even more rounds. Within a couple of weeks you may even complete the full 10 rounds in under 40 minutes. Always building, always improving. That's the key. Once you can successfully do 10 reps per round—Level 3—within the allotted time, you can hit the program.

The workouts in the program have the same basic structure as the test, only with more variety in the movements and five more minutes on the clock to complete them. You also get to choose which exercises you want to attempt from the Exercise Garage in Chapter 3. This keeps the workouts fresh and extends the life of the program. However, if you continually shuffle the workouts from day to day, it becomes more difficult to judge your progress. I suggest constructing three different workouts and sticking with them for at least one month. Each session write down the rounds completed and the time it took you, and every time you attempt the workout try to beat your previous score.

Each exercise in the circuit represents a type of basic movement pattern. You start with an upper-body movement such as a push-up or dip. Since your lower body is not directly involved in that exercise, you can immediately move into a leg-dominant task like a lunge or step-up. That's followed by a core-specific exercise, which includes gut-busters like V-ups. The last part of the round is a speed/cardio component that elevates the heart rate and improves endurance, such as donkey kicks or split-squat jumps.

By linking exercises in this order, you'll be able to work continuously with minimal rest to elicit the greatest metabolic disturbance. Substituting different exercises for each movement pattern means the variety of your workouts is limited only by your imagination. There are plenty of choices in the Exercise Garage, but I encourage you to seek out additional options from other resources.

Now, I know what you're thinking: Where are the biceps curls? What about triceps extensions? How am I going to burst my pipes? In due time. Those are solid isolation exercises, but not essential or a valuable use of your time at this stage of your development. I'm amazed every time I see someone overweight and out of shape spending a significant chunk of a gym session curling light dumbbells. What for? Attacking such a small muscle group will provide little help in trimming an expansive waistline. Curls can help define the biceps, but you've still got to strip fat from the body to show them off.

That's why we're sticking with the compound movements that work larger muscle groups. We need to build our race-car motor before worrying about the detailing. That will come later. Plus, those big movements will hit assistance muscles like the biceps and triceps anyway. You can't do a pull-up without the help of your biceps; no push-up or dip can be completed without involving the triceps. Trust me, no muscle will be neglected in this program.

Once you're able to consistently complete 10 rounds of 10 reps in under 45 minutes (see the three sample workouts on page 103), you can either move up to the intermediate-level workouts or continue to add more reps to each round. I know many people who are completely content to increase the reps or decrease their times in the beginning workouts, rather than move on to the intermediate program. Either they're not comfortable using weights, or they may have injuries that prevent them from doing so, and they get the muscular and cardiovascular results they're after from these workouts. They may appear simplistic, but they are that effective.

Still, if you're successful at this level, I encourage you not to stop. The intermediate workouts are likely to present a physical challenge unlike any you've ever faced. And you'll never know what you're truly capable of unless you're willing to do something you've never done before.

If you get proficient at the bodyweight exercises at this level, there are subtle ways to tweak them to enhance their difficulty without having to add any external load. Take the push-up. By positioning your hands farther outside or inside shoulder width, you create a more difficult movement—the former attacks the pecs, while the latter focuses more on the triceps. Or if you elevate your feet on a bench or box, it becomes a much tougher push-up, concentrating more on the upper pecs.

Same goes for the lunge. Elevate your back foot—commonly called the Bulgarian split-squat—and you'll increase the range of motion in the movement. Plus, the back foot can't provide as much assistance. As a result, the working leg gets a deeper, more intense contraction. Bulgarians must have solid oak legs because this subtle variation absolutely torches the quads.

You can also incorporate equipment found in most gyms as intensity amplifiers. For instance, resistance bands—thick, durable rubber bands made in varying widths to provide varying levels of resistance—are an inexpensive and highly useful way to increase the difficulty of certain movements without having to use weights. If you're doing push-ups, you can loop the ends around your thumbs and position the band across your back beneath your shoulder blades. Starting from the plank position, as you drop your chest to the floor—where you're weakest—the band will slacken and provide little additional resistance. As you push up, it will tighten and force you to work harder at the top of the movement, where you're strongest.

Or, when performing squats, you can loop the band under your feet and across your shoulders so that it's taut. As you drop into the squat, the band will slacken—just like when you're in the bottom of a push-up—and provide more resistance as you return to the standing position, the easiest part of the movement.

Suspension trainers, such as the TRX or Jungle Gym, are also effective ways to increase the difficulty of bodyweight movements. The instability of the straps makes exercises like push-ups and bodyweight rows more challenging, while also providing assistance for highly advanced moves like single-leg (pistol) squats. Add up all the possibilities and you see why so many trainers say one of the greatest pieces of exercise equipment people can use is staring right back at them in the mirror.

I started training with Donald six months after having my baby. I've been working out for most of my life and did so throughout my pregnancy. However, after delivery and getting back in the gym I wasn't seeing the results I wanted at the speed at which I wanted them with my previous trainer. My husband was working out with Donald and showing great progress in a short period of time, so I thought I'd give him a try.

I've never looked back.

What I like about Donald's workouts is that he combines weights with cardio so that you're constantly exerting yourself. You get stronger while you get leaner. He can determine your training level on the first day—not what you think your training level is—and cater the routines to push you without breaking you. Unlike other trainers who move clients through exercises to fill up an hour, Donald never looks at his watch. He creates a workout that day and there's no time limit for finishing it. It may take under an hour, it may take 1.5 hours. I like that the session is over only when the workout is done. All the while, Donald is right there, revving you up with his infectious energy.

I've also seen great results from his nutrition plan. I'm currently eating 1,400 calories a day, which is certainly less than I was accustomed to. He advocates clean foods—lean meats and fibrous vegetables—so you can eat a lot to stave off hunger without piling on the calories. I never feel starved or ravenous. Do I follow it seven days a week? No. But if I'm disciplined for five of those days I still get the outcome I want. That kind of flexibility makes it a diet I can stick to long-term.

Through the first six weeks' training with Donald I lost 10 pounds. Just to be able to sit in a pair of jeans after having a baby was awesome. The sacrifice in the gym and at the dinner table can be demanding, but the results are completely motivating. I can't say enough about Donald's training.

Monica Henshaw
Roanoke, Texas

45-MINUTE WORKOUT

		SAMPLE 1	LEVEL 1	LEVEL 2	LEVEL 3	LEVEL 4
		EXERCISES	REPS			
UPPER	1	FLOOR DIPS	6	8	10	12
LOWER	2	LUNGES	6	8	10	12
CORE	3	FULL SIT-UPS	6	8	10	12
CARDIO	4	SPLIT-SQUAT JUMPS	6	8	10	12

		SAMPLE 2	LEVEL 1	LEVEL 2	LEVEL 3	LEVEL 4
		EXERCISES	REPS			
UPPER	1	PUSH-UPS	6	8	10	12
LOWER	2	SQUATS	6	8	10	12
CORE	3	SUPERMAN	6	8	10	12
CARDIO	4	BURPEES	6	8	10	12

		SAMPLE 3	LEVEL 1	LEVEL 2	LEVEL 3	LEVEL 4
		EXERCISES	REPS			
UPPER	1	SHOULDER TAPS	6	8	10	12
LOWER	2	STEP-UPS	6	8	10	12
CORE	3	TOE TOUCHES	6	8	10	12
CARDIO	4	FROG THRUSTS	6	8	10	12

CHAPTER 5

THIRD GEAR

(INTERMEDIATE PROGRAM)

We are the change that we seek. —**Barack Obama**

This phase is for individuals who successfully completed the beginner workout plan or are coming to the book with an established base of strength and conditioning: dedicated gym-goers who have been training and lifting weights regularly for several years but need the push of a more sophisticated and intense fitness program. It's not for the faint of heart—I honestly believe it's more challenging than what many books and programs offer as advanced training. If there's any indecision about whether you're ready, I recommend attempting the Level 3 workout of the beginner program to be sure you're capable of handling this increased workload. The worst thing that can happen is that you spend a week getting familiar with this style of training and establishing a solid base to build from. A win-win from my perspective.

Compared to the beginner workouts, the intermediate workouts kick up the volume of training and complexity of movements. You'll still be performing full-body routines three days a week, with a day off between workouts. You'll need the rest to get acclimated to the added stresses provided by the dumbbell and kettlebell movements introduced here that accompany some of the bodyweight movements you performed as a beginner. The addition of free weights increases resistance to bolster strength and exact a greater metabolic toll as well as preserve and build muscle mass, whereas steady-state, traditional cardiovascular activity—running on the hamster wheel—is actually catabolic and breaks down muscle. Numerous studies have shown that resistance training in conjunction with a proper diet is far superior for fat loss and body composition than steady-state cardio. Wiry, long-distance runners work out in steady-state conditions; muscular sprinters do resistance training to build explosive power. Which type of body do you want? And the great thing about dumbbells and kettlebells is that even if you're not that familiar with them, they're relatively safe and easy to use.

Just as with the beginner program, you will have a maximum time allotment of 45 minutes to complete a workout. However, instead of four movements performed back-to-back for each round, there are additional upper-body, lower-body, and speed/cardio exercises, for a total of seven. That's right, nearly double the workload. Like I said, this will definitely test you. For that reason, it's wise to start back at 6 reps per exercise and gradually increase with success. Don't worry if you can't make the full 10 rounds or 45 minutes in your first few attempts. Again, these are goals to shoot for that you may not always reach. The key is to not give up and to continually strive to improve. However, if you fail to complete a workout three consecutive times, you should lessen the load by scaling back either the number of reps or the amount of weight used for each exercise.

As you will see in the sample workouts on pages 112–113, the movements are arranged in an order that moves the target areas of work around the body in a noncompeting fashion. You will start out with an upper-body pushing movement, followed by a lower-body quad-dominant exercise. As the upper body is tested, the lower half rests, and vice versa. Then you will perform a speed component that often requires full-body interaction but no additional resistance. After that, it's back to the upper body, only this time it's a pulling movement to work the back of the body. Then a hip-dominant lower-body exercise to work the posterior chain, followed by another speed element, with a core movement finishing the round. The design is structured to allow the most possible continuous movement to create the biggest metabolic demand. Rest should be taken as needed. If you're unfamiliar with this type of training, it can be a big ask. So don't be a hero: work at a reasonable clip.

For example, let's say you're attempting 6 reps per exercise, and it takes roughly 30 seconds to complete a set. To be on the conservative side we'll allow for some transition time between exercises and give an approximate estimate of 4 minutes per round. That means if you're doing dumbbell bench presses as your upper-body pushing movement, it will be about 4 minutes between sets. The cardiovascular demand of shuffling between the seven movements will test your lungs, but the muscle groups involved—your pecs, shoulders, and triceps—should have plenty of rest between applications. And if you manage that exact pace for the full 10 rounds, you'll complete the workout with 5 minutes to spare.

Once you're able to complete 10 rounds of 10 reps in the allotted time, you can either add more weight to the exercises or add more reps. Or you can choose to move up to the advanced program. The addition of barbell training, more technical movements, and dedicated strength days of the advanced program may not be attractive to everybody. Or you might be working out at home and have only a set of adjustable dumbbells at your disposal. Not a problem. If you're content with the intermediate program, the variability in resistance and exercise structure makes it extremely adaptable and effective long-term. I've shown these workouts to serious strength athletes, and many balk at the level of conditioning it takes to complete them. Keep switching up the movements, adding weight, and breaking personal best times in these workouts and you can use this program indefinitely.

WEIGHT SELECTION

Choosing the right poundage on movements is critical for getting the most out of this style of training. It's much better to err on the side of too light of a weight than too heavy. Don't forget that your goal is to complete 10 rounds of 10 reps. If you're accustomed to doing 3×10 shoulder presses with 40-pound dumbbells, you may need to drop down to a pair of 25-pounders, to have a chance to finish—and more important—while maintaining good form.

An experienced lifter may look at this program and think, "Three days a week? That's not enough. I work out more than that now." But I'm betting you don't work out quite like this. Believe me, this type of training will take a toll. Allow your body time to recover between workouts. Don't overdo it by performing the workouts on consecutive days or by squeezing in a fourth one during the same week. Sometimes less is more. Your muscles are stimulated in the gym, but they grow during recovery. Allow them the chance. Plus, if you continually dominate and complete 10 rounds of the intermediate workouts, feel free to take the challenge of the advanced level.

That said, I can appreciate someone's desire to stay active as much as possible. Not too many days go by where I don't break a sweat. But you don't always have to be in the gym slinging weights. Play a sport, ride a bike, go for a run, swim, take a yoga or Pilates class. When we hit forty and cross into middle age, we start to encounter noticeable loss in our mobility—sitting at a desk hunched over a computer all day doesn't help—and our joints get more affected by repetitive movement like constant exercise. Ask your body to perform in all different types of motion and activities. It's not only beneficial from a physical standpoint, it keeps you from being a slave to the gym. At least one day a week you're sure to find me on a basketball court somewhere. It's a great competitive outlet that also allows me to judge whether my workouts are making a difference in my athletic performance. Mostly, though, it's a wonderful release of pure, childlike enjoyment that's good for the body and even better for the mind.

I know some guys get turned off by this. Why should they use less weight than they're capable of using? More weight equals more gains, right? I'm asking you to leave your ego in the locker room. Don't get so concerned with how much weight you're lifting. Your muscles don't know the number of pounds in your hand, only whether the weight is providing the necessary stimulus for growth. And trust me, these workouts will get you bigger and stronger. Besides the personal experiences of me and my trainees, there's actual evidence to back this strategy up. A study published in the *Journal of Applied Physiology* several years ago revealed that weight lifters who took 3 sets to failure with 30 percent of their 1-rep max—the most weight they could lift in an exercise for 1 repetition—achieved muscle growth equal to that of lifters who took 3 sets to failure with 80 percent of their 1-rep max. It took the 30 percent group more reps to reach muscular failure, but the gains were still the same. The big meatheads at your gym who bust the veins in their neck moving stacks of iron will disagree, but you don't need to lift exceedingly heavy weight to build muscle.

Plus, if you start out with 25-pound dumbbells on your shoulder presses and a few weeks later you're up to 30-pounders, you're getting stronger. If a few weeks after that you're still using 30 pounds, but you've gone from 8 to 10 reps a set, you're getting stronger. If you manage to shave a few minutes off your workout time while using the same weight and rep scheme, you're getting stronger. Notice a pattern? Keep progressing, keep getting better each workout, and the results will come. Before long you'll be in the best shape of your life and those meatheads will still be clanking iron over their big fat bellies.

Training has been a real journey for me. Ten years ago I was out of shape, leading a predominantly sedentary lifestyle. I didn't like the path I was headed down and adopted the fallback plan most people turn to in my situation: I joined a big-box gym and took classes. When that proved unsatisfying, I adopted plan B: enlisting the help of one of the gym's personal trainers. Again, the results proved disappointing.

Then I discovered weights. I absolutely love them and what they do for my body. Anyone who thinks weight lifting makes you bulky and inflexible hasn't spent much time using them properly. Adding weight training to my regimen made a marked difference in my conditioning and appearance, which I would never have imagined when I first began working out.

But something changed about 18 months ago. For some reason, no matter how little I ate, or how much I trained, I kept putting on weight. And because I kept working out, the excess weight did a number on my joints, including a severe case of plantar fasciitis. I was in pain, and I was overweight. Ironically, I was trying to get ultralean at the time, having adopted a drastically low 20-carbs-a-day diet. That ill-advised eating approach, along with now being in my midforties, caused a hormonal imbalance that precipitated my weight spike.

That's when Donald stepped in. I belonged to his gym and had been taking group classes with one of his partners, John Simon. Donald saw that I was struggling and asked if he could help. He determined that consistently living in a substantial caloric deficit was causing my body to store fat, and I needed to adjust my eating habits—small tweaks to the timing and portion sizes as well as the nutritional content of my food intake. So instead of ingesting practically nothing leading into a workout, I started having a significant breakfast well before hitting the gym. My meals also became more balanced, as I no longer shunned carbs.

I also began training one-on-one with Donald. I really gravitated toward his detail-oriented approach. He understands that everybody responds differently to certain types of training and caters the workouts to the individual. As someone who has done CrossFit, Donald knows I like to train with heavy weights, but he makes sure I balance my gym time with cardio, light weights, high-intensity intervals, and even bodyweight exercises. I absolutely love the variety.

He's also incredibly encouraging and motivating. Some trainers feel the need to scream to inspire, but Donald is always upbeat and positive. At the same time, he never allows you to skate through a workout. He knows you're there to see change—more muscle, less fat, improved conditioning—and will make sure you never cheat yourself.

After the first six months of training with Donald I lost 12 pounds. More important, there was a noticeable shift in the amount of muscle on my body and how I looked. Best of all, I've never felt in better shape. I'm just very grateful for Donald's help and look forward to seeing him every day. He's been a real godsend on my journey to a healthier life.

Gina Mullen
Bartonville, Texas

3 DAYS A WEEK
COMPLETE AS MANY ROUNDS AS YOU CAN FOR 45 MIN.

IF YOU COMPLETE 10 OR MORE ROUNDS, ADD WEIGHT OR REPS

| | EXERCISES | WEIGHT | 6 REPS | | 8 REPS | | 10 REPS | | |
			DAY	ROUNDS	DAY	ROUNDS	DAY	ROUNDS	
UPPER	DB BENCH PRESS								
LOWER	GOBLET SQUAT								
SPE	KB/DB SWING								INCREASE WEIGHT
UPPER	DB ROW								
LOWER	DB LUNGES								
SPE	DB UP-DOWN								
CORE	FULL SIT-UPS								

| | EXERCISES | WEIGHT | 6 REPS | | 8 REPS | | 10 REPS | | |
			DAY	ROUNDS	DAY	ROUNDS	DAY	ROUNDS	
UPPER	DB SHOULDER PRESS								
LOWER	DB DEAD LIFT								
SPE	DB THRUSTER								INCREASE WEIGHT
UPPER	DB UPRIGHT ROWS								
LOWER	DB STEP-UPS								

				6 REPS		8 REPS		10 REPS		
SPE	SUMO DEADLIFT HIGH-PULL									
CORE	ALTERNATING V-UPS									
		WEIGHT	DAY	ROUNDS	DAY	ROUNDS	DAY	ROUNDS		
	EXERCISES									
UPPER	DB INCLINE PRESS									INCREASE WEIGHT
LOWER	GOBLET SQUAT									
SPE	KB SNATCH (EACH ARM)									
UPPER	FRONT RAISE									
LOWER	DB RDL									
SPE	RENEGADE ROW									
CORE	TOE TOUCHES									

CHAPTER 6

FIFTH GEAR

(ADVANCED PROGRAM)

Impossible is not a fact. It's an opinion. Impossible is not a declaration. It's a dare. Impossible is potential. Impossible is temporary. Impossible is nothing. —**Muhammad Ali**

If you have to ask if this program is right for you, you're probably not ready. It's strictly for dedicated individuals who have already made training and proper nutrition a significant part of their lives. If you don't already have that base to build from, these workouts will be overwhelming. You've got to be a beast to take them down.

The setups mirror the same routines that I perform with the top athletes at my gym on a weekly basis. It's four workouts a week—two for hypertrophy and conditioning and two that are more power- and strength-based. So unlike the beginner and intermediate programs, you will be training on consecutive days. There's a significant amount of barbell work and the introduction of more intricate movements, such as Olympic lifts. Because the weights get heavier, and the moves more challenging, technique becomes even more pivotal. If you're unfamiliar with some of these exercises, it may seem intimidating at first. I encourage you to go slow. Get acclimated to the movements before adding lots of weight. The tutorials in the Exercise Garage will certainly help, and I encourage you to seek out guidance from a certified trainer who specializes in these types of lifts. If you're willing to take on these workouts, shift into fifth gear and give them everything you've got. I promise you unprecedented results.

The format of the hypertrophy and conditioning workouts is similar to the intermediate program. You will have a maximum of 45 minutes to complete a workout consisting of a seven-exercise circuit of varying movement patterns in a 6- to 10-rep range done for up to 10 rounds. Unlike the intermediate program, though, the workouts are more body-part-specific. For instance, the first workout of the week has no dedicated lower-body work, replacing both of those exercises with a power movement at the beginning of the circuit and an additional core exercise. This is done so that when you perform the strength-focused lower-body workout the following day, your legs are still relatively fresh. After a day off you would perform another muscle-building and conditioning circuit, only this time with a lower-body emphasis. This would save your upper body for the strength-based workout that finishes the week. As with the previous two levels, you can choose from the Exercise Garage in Chapter 3 to construct your own program. The sample workouts on pages 120–121 will help spell everything out.

STRENGTH DAYS

Besides the power movements and the more sophisticated barbell movements, the big addition in the advanced program is the dedicated strength days. These are designed for you to move serious weight—slap some plates on the bar, grit your teeth, and see what you're made of. The workout is still a maximum of 45 minutes or 10 rounds, but the circuit is composed of only four movements: a power exercise, two body-part-specific lifts (upper or lower), and a speed element. The rep range also decreases to 3 to 5 reps per set. So there are fewer movements, less volume, and much more time available between sets. Which means the weight used goes up.

WAY UP.

To see what I mean, let's take a look at Day 2 from the sample week on page 120. The exercises are a Kettlebell Snatch (power), DB Lunge, Deadlift (lower), and

Kettlebell Swing (speed). If you opt to do 3 reps per exercise, I would suggest starting with a weight you can lift for at least 5 reps. You can always increase the weight if it's not challenging enough. Since the KB Snatch would be 3 reps per arm and DB lunges 3 reps per leg, the total amount of reps for each round would be 18. That's not a lot. Your actual work time for each round should be 45–60 seconds. But the point here is not muscular and cardiovascular endurance; it's to concentrate on increasing strength and power output through heavy compound movements. As long as you pace yourself properly—once again, rest as needed—you will have plenty of time to recover from lifting more substantial loads.

Just as with the muscle-building, fat-burning circuits, monitoring performance in each strength workout is a must. Whether adding weight to the bar, adding more reps to the exercises, or performing the exercises in less time, you're still looking to improve work capacity from the previous session. Knowledge is power—I recommend using the charts provided in this book, but you're free to use a notebook, app, or whatever kind of stat-keeping device you prefer. But make sure you know and are constantly challenging your previous personal bests. That's how to continually build raw strength and power.

TOOLS OF THE TRADE

Not only are the advanced workouts demanding to do—I mean it, this program is '85 Bears defense tough—they're also a little tricky to set up. Performing a 45-minute circuit that requires the use of multiple Olympic bars, a deadlifting platform, heavy kettlebells, and box jumps may be too much for the average gym to handle. Unless you've outfitted a complete home gym, you may need to seek out a training facility with the necessary space and equipment to accommodate these workouts.

You can also make equipment substitutions when necessary to make a workout feasible. For instance, if you have access to only one Olympic bar, you can use dumb-bell movements for the other resistance exercises. Or you can use kettlebells when doing some of the power moves such as the clean or the snatch. However, you'll only

Having played with two all-time great quarterbacks—Brett Favre and Aaron Rodgers—I'm often asked which one I think is better. It's a tough question. Like trying to decide which is your favorite child. The truth is both were awesome to play with and had their own unique styles. Brett was the ultimate gunslinger, always looking to make a big play downfield. Even if a receiver was double-covered, he believed his arm strength could get him the ball. Aaron was more deliberate. If a receiver was covered, he immediately moved on to his next option. He'd take what the defense gave him and methodically pick them apart. If needed, both guys would take off running to move the chains and keep a drive alive. In other words, you could win with either guy behind center, and that's why both quarterbacked winning teams in the Super Bowl.

Same goes for barbells and dumbbells. People like to draw comparisons and distinctions over which is more effective. Don't worry about it. Both have their strengths when it comes to training—you can lift more total weight with a barbell; you work unilaterally and get a better range of motion with dumbbells—and both can get the job done. That's why I always tell trainees it shouldn't be an either/or situation. Get the best of both worlds.

be limiting yourself in the long run by setting boundaries on what you're able to accomplish based solely on access to the right environment.

A lot of books or training systems are proud to offer alternatives to make things more convenient for their users, but I don't consider convenience one of the main requirements of an advanced training program. Convenience is a shortcut. Convenience is the path of least resistance. Convenience is how people get out of shape in the first place. I expect athletes, especially those at an advanced level, to take ownership of their training and do what's necessary to achieve their goals. This program takes real commitment, from maximum effort in the gym right down to where you work out. That's the dedication and determination required to construct the ultimate sports-car body. It's tough and takes sacrifice. But if it were easy, everybody would be walking around with broad shoulders and tree-trunk thighs.

When lifting heavy, one of the tricks of the trade is to employ full-body tension. What do I mean by that? Watch the biggest guys at your gym trying to bench or squat hundreds of pounds; every part of their bodies, from head to toe, is involved in the lift. Every muscle is squeezed, and there's not a single area that is lax or disengaged. Doesn't matter if it's a biceps curl: they're involving their glutes, quads, and chest to help move the weight.

The best way to discover how to recruit every power source is to think of your body as one big, connected unit. You want tension running through every inch of it. When some part of your body is not firing, energy is being lost. That missing energy is power that could be used to move the weight. And when you're trying to move heavy weights, every ounce of force counts.

Take the bench press. With the chest, shoulders, and triceps as the prime movers in the exercise, most inexperienced lifters rely strictly on those muscles. Their feet are placed casually on the floor, their cores aren't engaged, their hands have a relaxed grip on the bar, and their lats aren't contracted. Sure, they can still move the weight. But not with the force they could be generating if their feet were screwed into the floor, their core was tight, they put a death grip on the bar, and their shoulder blades were retracted to create a more powerful pushing platform. Now the whole body is working to move the weight.

Same goes for a lower-body-dominant lift like the squat. Again, everybody is consumed with using the legs to lower themselves down and then push themselves away from the floor. But the experienced lifter knows that his core must be also stiff as a board, his shoulders pulled back and tight, and his grip on the bar turning his knuckles white. That creates the full-body tension needed to crank out reps with heavy weights. Otherwise energy will bleed from the movement, you won't lift as much weight as you could, and you'll be in danger of getting stapled to the floor. Next time you hit the gym, give it a try. I bet you'll notice an immediate difference.

4 DAYS A WEEK
COMPLETE AS MANY ROUNDS AS YOU CAN FOR 45 MIN.

DAY 1			6 REPS		8 REPS		10 REPS		
	EXERCISES	WEIGHT	DAY	ROUNDS	DAY	ROUNDS	DAY	ROUNDS	
POWER	POWER CLEAN								
UPPER	DB BENCH PRESS								INCREASE WEIGHT
SPE	BURPEE								
CORE	STRAIGHT-LEG SIT-UPS								
UPPER	PUSH-UP								
SPE	KB SWING								
CORE	FULL SIT-UP								

DAY 2 DESIGNED TO BE A STRENGTH DAY—MOVE WEIGHT!			3 REPS		4 REPS		5 REPS		
	EXERCISES	WEIGHT	DAY	ROUNDS	DAY	ROUNDS	DAY	ROUNDS	
POWER	KB SNATCH (EACH ARM)								INCREASE WEIGHT
LOWER	DB LUNGE								
LOWER	DEADLIFT								
SPE	KB SWING								

DAY 3 OFF

DAY 4			6 REPS		8 REPS		10 REPS		
	EXERCISES	WEIGHT	DAY	ROUNDS	DAY	ROUNDS	DAY	ROUNDS	
POWER	BOX JUMPS (REPS)								INCREASE WEIGHT
LOWER	BACK SQUAT								
SPE	FROG THRUSTS								
CORE	ALTERNATING V-UPS								
LOWER	BB RDL								
SPE	DONKEY KICKS								
CORE	RENEGADE ROW								

DAY 5 DESIGNED TO BE A STRENGTH DAY—MOVE WEIGHT!			3 REPS		4 REPS		5 REPS		
	EXERCISES	WEIGHT	DAY	ROUNDS	DAY	ROUNDS	DAY	ROUNDS	
POWER	POWER CLEAN								INCREASE WEIGHT
UPPER	BENCH PRESS								
UPPER	SHOULDER PRESS								
SPE	BURPEE								

DISCIP
TO EAT

LINED
CLEAN

NUTRITION OVERVIEW

Exercise is your king, and nutrition is your queen. Together they create your fitness kingdom. —**Jack LaLanne**

There are decisions in our lives that define us. When I was in college I met my wife, Tina. At the time I was also still dealing drugs. While it was stupid to jeopardize my scholarship and (more important) my freedom, it was putting money in my pocket. I never used, only profited. But when Tina found out, she gave me an ultimatum: selling drugs or her. The street life was all the men of my family knew—that was how we survived. We didn't think about our future beyond the next day. So, ridiculous as it may seem in retrospect, at the time I was tempted to let Tina walk out of my life.

I THANK GOD EVERY DAY I DID NOT.

She put me on a righteous path and got me to focus on school and athletics. She supported my career every step of the way and became the rock of our family. She is simply my everything. I just could not imagine my life without her. In fact, I'd probably already be six feet under.

Not every decision carries such personal consequences. Sometimes we're forced into making difficult job-related choices. I remember in 2000 I had an opportunity to try for a medal in the Summer Olympics, competing in the high jump. I brought it up with the Packers general manager and he said I could either play in the NFL or go for the gold—couldn't have both. Again, I think I chose wisely.

Right now I'm presenting you with an important lifestyle choice: you can continue to freely eat whatever you want, whenever you want, or you can start to be disciplined about your nutrition. You can take seriously the ramifications of your food choices and what it means to your future. It may not have the importance of picking the right spouse, but it's not far behind.

If the goal of this book is to turn your body into a finely tuned sports car, you're going to need the right workouts to enhance the exterior, and, just as important, the proper nutrients to fuel the engine. The two elements go hand in hand—the body is made in the gym and defined in the kitchen; resistance training breaks down muscles and the food you feed it builds them back up. The higher quality the workout program and the nutrition used to power it, the better the body looks and performs.

A great deal of misinformation clouds books, magazines, and websites when it comes to healthy eating, weight management, and working out. They make it seem like a foreign language that can be mastered only by a chosen few, a secret code that takes wizardry to decipher. The prospect of losing weight and toning up is confusing and overwhelms people into thinking that doing right by their bodies is exceedingly complicated. They think it's too arduous, too time-consuming, and too expensive. That's why all the "get fit quick" systems are so appealing. They're not a big investment, and if they don't work—or work only temporarily—it's not a big loss. And it only reaffirms what the user believed in the first place: getting in shape is too difficult. It's not. But discipline, smarts, and even a little imagination are required.

Start with this: close your eyes and think of a brand-new shiny black Porsche (that's my favorite car, but you're welcome to choose your own model). Shimmering in the sun, fully detailed, with fresh tires, fine upholstery, and a full tank of premium gas, this car is ready for the ride of its life. After all, it's in perfect shape. Even if it's a slightly used model with some miles on it, proper care and maintenance has kept it in pristine condition and ready for the road ahead.

Now take a minute and compare your body to that car. Does it possess a strong, durable frame with impeccable insides, always filled with the right fuel and fluids? Or instead of a Porsche, maybe you're envisioning an old Pinto? Not to worry if you feel like a junker right now; looking and performing like a Porsche is definitely in your future.

But, contrary to what a lot of books claim, building a body does not happen overnight. As I mentioned earlier, it's created by doing small things consistently over time. You've just read what it takes to build a sports-car body and engine in the gym. From a nutrition perspective, it means putting the proper foods, fluids, and nutrients into your body on a regular basis. Like the car, you would not put cheap gas in it and expect it to run at its optimal level. So why would you fuel your body with low-quality food and expect it to be at its best?

It's no wonder most people are confused by the concept of proper nutrition. They read fad-diet books, eyeball the covers of magazines, and listen to the latest celebrity weight-loss trends, all to be left in a maze of distorted possibilities. Some sell the fool's gold that a Pinto can be converted to a Porsche in a couple of months. Others paint a picture of painstaking dedication that can be accomplished only by fitness zealots who spend all day obsessing over each carrot shaving in their salads. The truth is it's not nearly that confusing, and the good news is that any car, regardless of condition, can be refurbished.

At its most practical level, food is simply the fuel that makes our bodies run. The better fuel we put in them, the better performance we get out of them, and the longer they run. However, most people have grown to view food as an indulgence to be explored at every feeding. They view meals as opportunities to eat whatever they want, as much as they want it.

Breaking this pattern becomes even more important (and difficult) as we hit middle age. Our metabolism slows, our activity level lessens, and those high-calorie, low-nutrient meals do increasingly more damage to our waistlines—unlike an actual car there's no value in our bodies having a spare tire—and overall health. It's not easy, but you can make the transition if you really want to.

In my ninth season with the Packers I had to make a conversion from flanker, or split end, to slot receiver. A flanker generally lines up near the sideline and uses his speed and athleticism to blow by defensive backs to make big plays. When I broke into the league I was a track star with great leaping ability. Like a young kid who could eat whatever he wanted and not gain weight, I could rely on my natural talents to succeed. Now I was a veteran with lots of NFL wear and tear on my legs, and we had younger receivers more suited to work the outside of the field. If I still wanted to earn a paycheck, I had to shift to the slot and work the middle of the field more. It's a position that requires toughness and smarts. You have to know how to spot holes in the defense and then protect yourself from collisions with massive linebackers and strong safeties with bad intentions. I was learning a new role that didn't come naturally, but it made me a better receiver.

Your eating habits need to evolve as well, taking an almost utilitarian approach to consuming the proper carbohydrates, proteins, fats, and fluids on a daily basis. The occasional cheat is permitted, but the large majority of meals constitute clean foods—high in nutrition, low in junk. However, that type of discipline is where so many people give up. Instead of eating to live, they live to eat. And proper nutrition is not nearly as much fun as eating whatever you want, whenever you want it.

But how much do you value your body? If you got only one car your entire life, I bet you'd take pretty meticulous care of it. I'd bet you'd prefer it be a Porsche rather than a Pinto. Well, we get only one body. And the truth is that nutrition and eating properly is not that difficult, nor does it have to be boring and predictable. Yes, a few key ingredients should be implemented on a daily basis to eat healthy for a lifetime. It takes discipline to make sure those ingredients are respected. It takes self-control to make sure indulgences are minimized. Yet what may seem like sacrifice results in a trimmer waistline, improved health, and more energy to do what you want to do, whether that's hitting the gym, playing soccer with your kids, or simply living every day to its fullest.

The nutrition component of this book is designed to help put you in the driver's seat of your health and future. The following chapters provide all the basic education and know-how you'll need to turbocharge your diet and dominate your workouts. You'll learn to value the calories you consume more than to solely satisfy hunger. Choosing meals and snacks based on convenience and pleasing taste without regard for quantity or ingredients is like filling your Porsche with low-octane sludge. Not only will your engine sputter, but your sports-car chassis will look more like that Pinto you're looking to replace. Instead, I'm going to show you simple but proven methods for nutrition that spur lasting physical change. You'll discover that it's actually easy to cultivate eating habits that greatly improve your energy levels, performance, and appearance. Get ready—your Porsche is about to take off.

CHAPTER 7
FUELING THE TANK

It's not about low carb; it's about low crap.

Carbohydrates are to our bodies what gas is to a car—they give us the energy to operate. Recent fad diets and media distortion have demonized carbs. There's a perception that they make people fat and should be severely curtailed, or consumed only under certain circumstances. I've heard nutty suggestions such as you should never eat carbs after 6 p.m.; or our bodies are incapable of digesting grains; or you should save your carbs just for days with a full moon—an exaggeration, but you get the point.

The reality is carbohydrates are vital macronutrients (meaning they provide calories) that give us energy over the course of the day to live, think, run, jump, lift, and be active. In fact, your brain and central nervous system's preferred source of fuel is carbohydrate. If you're an athlete, carbs are indispensable. I've read numerous accounts that claim the body can more optimally run with fat as the primary fuel source—using ketones instead of glucose—but I've also personally seen too many people struggling in the gym and miserable in life with this model. Limiting yourself to extremely low levels of carbs deprives the body of countless micronutrients, not to mention dramatically decreases performance and energy levels. I also believe there's a negative psychological impact of never allowing yourself to enjoy the occasional carb-rich food. Life is too short to eat bunless burgers with no French fries.

The "problem" with carbs—as with any food really—is when you eat too many of them, particularly the sweeter, more processed varieties. You know, the junk that comes in a box and expires in two years. Just as you wouldn't top off a gas tank that is already full, eating excess carbs, or more than the body needs based on your activity level, can start to add inches to your waistline. Active, more muscular people burn a lot of energy and need more carbs to replenish what was used; sedentary people expend less energy and don't require as frequent refueling. (What's worse is that all those desk jockeys often have a top-drawer stash of candy or junk food.) The category of carbohydrates and the timing of their ingestion is also of critical importance. As long as you're educated on the effects of different types of carbs and base your consumption of them on need and activity level rather than desire—this is where discipline becomes critical—there's no drawback to including them as an integral part of your diet.

SIMPLE CARBOHYDRATES

Just as there are different grades of gas, there are different types of carbohydrates. Simple carbohydrates are made up of monosaccharides and disaccharides, which are one- and two-part sugar molecules. Because they are so small, the body can break them down faster. For exercise this can be a great thing, as simple carbs can provide fast energy to the body to continue exertion. For example, sipping a sports drink during a rigorous workout is like stopping for small amounts of gas every few miles on a trip; it keeps your tank from running low. It's not an excuse to guzzle a six-pack of Gatorade, but under these circumstances, simple sugar is helpful as it is being used up quickly to fuel the body.

However, consuming large amounts of simple carbohydrates throughout the day has drawbacks. It can cause your blood sugar to dramatically spike, followed by a significant drop. As your blood sugar level rides this roller coaster, so too does your energy level—one minute you feel great, the next you're hitting the couch for a nap. In order to prevent that energy-lull feeling, most people look for another simple carbohydrate like candy, cookies, or soda to give them more energy to escape the blood sugar slump. The problem is that sooner rather than later, this crash will come again.

Think about sitting at your desk at work at 2:30 and needing that afternoon pick-me-up. You reach for a candy bar, bag of chips, or snack food and maybe wash it down with a soft drink or sugary coffee concoction. You get a quick boost of energy, followed by the inevitable crash. Worse yet, you're back at the vending machine at 4:00 looking for another sugar rush to get you through the day—the vicious simple-carb cycle continues. Your body's gas tank is ping-ponging back and forth from full to empty and you're not even burning any fuel. But consuming tons of unwanted calories? You'd better believe it.

SIMPLE CARBOHYDRATE LIST

Table sugar

Honey and agave nectar

Corn and maple syrup

Candy

Cookies, cakes, and other pastries

Soda

Fruit and fruit drinks

White flour

FRUIT

Depending on who you ask, nature's candy toes the line between sweet treat and dietary staple. Compared to many vegetables—their brethren in the produce aisle—and other whole foods, fruits tend to be higher in sugar, particularly fructose (fruit sugar), which when consumed in excess can have negative effects. It's not to say you can't or shouldn't eat fruit, but like any food, there are appropriate amounts. Some diets misrepresent fruit by calling certain varieties like bananas and grapes "sugary," putting them in the simple-carb category, and slot their consumption solely around workouts or the occasional treat. On the other hand, options like berries and apples, which have lower sugar and higher fiber contents, are viewed more as complex carbs and can be eaten more frequently.

But I always give a green light to eating all kinds of fruit because they are nutrient-rich. Where fructose can become an issue is as an added sugar in soft drinks and other processed foods. But that's not the case in a whole food like fruit. Plus, fruit has a high water content, helping hydrate the body, and contains fiber, vitamins, minerals, and other phytonutrients that are beneficial to good health. As far as snacks go you could do a lot worse than a piece of fruit.

Still, if you're concerned about your waistline you need to be cognizant of how much sugar you're consuming, be it from fruit or other foods high in sugar. While they are nutrient-rich, fruit contains calories. Given the sweet taste and solid reputation—I'm touting it right now—it's easy to get carried away. Like anything else, sensible portion sizing still applies. Slicing a banana into your oatmeal at breakfast is nothing to worry about; having the entire bunch throughout the day can easily trip up your weight-loss ambitions.

Which makes it key to know the appropriate serving sizes. One fruit serving is roughly 15 grams of carbohydrate. As you'll note from the following list, these servings can add up quickly if you're not disciplined. Sit in front of the TV with a bowl of grapes and it's not difficult to reach the bottom. Depending on your weight-loss goals, stick to two to four servings per day and you'll be in good shape (literally).

- One baseball-size fruit (apple, pear, peach, orange, etc.)
- ½ banana
- ½ cup chopped fruit (pineapple, melons, mango, etc.)
- ¾ cup berries
- ¼ cup dried fruit (raisins, Craisins, etc.)
- 15 bite-size fruits like grapes or cherries
- 4 oz. 100% fruit juice

COMPLEX CARBOHYDRATES

The better alternative to loading up on simple carbs is to power your body with complex carbohydrates the majority of the day. As their name implies, these carbs are more intricate—they contain molecules and molecules of glucose (sugar), starch, and fiber—and break down gradually, to provide a steadier flow of energy and stave off hunger. Although not as tasty as many simple carbs—you won't find a lot of complex carbs on the dessert menu—they are generally a healthier option.

Plus, the fiber found in complex carbohydrates is dietary gold. There are two kinds. Insoluble fiber is like a broom—it works to promote gastrointestinal motility by sweeping out the garbage and keeping you regular. This type of fiber is found in vegetables, whole wheat, bran, and foods made from those grains. Soluble fiber, on the other hand, can bind to cholesterol, helping to lower total and LDL (bad cholesterol) levels in the body. Examples of soluble fiber include oats, nuts, seeds, legumes, and fruit where you can eat the skin like apples, pears, and berries. And since fiber doesn't digest, it travels through the body "pushing stuff" through the digestive tract, helping you feel full faster and maintaining that satiety longer. It staves off hunger and keeps your plumbing working—so find yourself some fiber.

COMPLEX CARBOHYDRATE LIST

Whole grains:

Whole wheat, oats, quinoa, couscous, farro, barley, buckwheat, brown rice, and so on

Starchy vegetables:

Potato, sweet potato/yams, corn, peas, winter squash (butternut, acorn, and spaghetti squash), pumpkin

Beans and legumes

Vegetables

The grain portion of complex carbohydrates such as breads, pastas, rice, and oats provide more grams of carbohydrate per serving than foods like vegetables and beans. Thanks to the media and loudmouths in the carb-phobe community, these foods have been particularly maligned over the past few years as being fat-inducing, illness-causing, and utterly avoidable. There's even a school of thought that the human body isn't capable of digesting them. The thinking goes that humans evolved walking the Earth millions of years ago existing on meat, vegetables, nuts, certain fruits, and seeds. That's what the body thrives on. Not noodles. I'm not educated enough in biological anthropology to speak to the theory's validity, but I do know that whole grains are rich in B vitamins, iron, fiber, and other phytonutrients that help my body fight off illnesses and stay strong, not to mention help it recover from strenuous workouts. And when I don't eat them, I die at the gym and am pretty cranky and edgy—the definition of a lose-lose proposition. Plus, I know many fit and healthy people who eat whole-grain bread, oatmeal, quinoa, and brown rice on a regular basis. Again, portion size is key, as overeating grains, just like any other food group, can lead to weight gain if you consume more than your body needs for its activity level.

Vegetables, on the other hand, contain some grams of carbohydrate but are much higher in fiber. In fact, vegetables are really like a "free food" provided they are not slathered with butter, cream, or cheese sauce. You will get sick of eating vegetables before you can eat too many calories from them due to their high water and fiber content. I dare you to try to gain weight on roasted kale. Starchy vegetables (listed earlier) contain more carbohydrate than broccoli or spinach, so count them more like a grain on the carbohydrate scale. They are nutrient-dense and healthy for you so definitely eat them; just be aware of the portion size.

Here are some easy ways to include more veggies in meals and snacks:

- Raw veggies dipped in a few tablespoons of hummus
- Spinach or kale blended into a smoothie
- Baby carrots dipped in 1 to 2 Tbsp. peanut butter

- Mix vegetables into common recipes that your family already enjoys
- Try shredding or spiraling vegetables to use instead of pasta in dishes like spaghetti and lasagna, and mash cauliflower instead of potatoes

The key to carbohydrate success is eating adequate amounts of grains and fruit (our meal plans will help you determine what that is for you), filling up on nonstarchy vegetables at meals and snacks, and saving those simple carbs for special occasions.

CARB-COUNTING CHART

Food	Grams of Carbohydrate	Portion Size Example
1 slice bread	15 grams	Cassette tape
½ cup cooked grain	25 to 30 grams	Lightbulb
1 small potato	25 to 30 grams	Computer mouse
1 cup cereal, rice, pasta	45 grams	Baseball

LOWER-CALORIE CARBOHYDRATE SWAPS

Carbohydrate Food	Lower-Calorie Swap
Biscuit	English muffin
Bagel	2 slices whole-wheat bread or 2 corn tortillas
Sugary cereal	Oatmeal
1 cup pasta	1 cup spiraled squash and zucchini
1 cup mashed potatoes	Mashed cauliflower
French fries	Roasted sweet potato wedges
Chips	Whole-wheat crackers or baked pita chips

ADDED SUGARS

You expect certain foods like candy, cake, and ice cream to contain high sugar counts. That's why they're referred to as "sweets." However, what has become alarmingly prevalent in the American diet is the inclusion of added sugars and starches in foods you wouldn't expect—bread, barbecue sauce, fruit-flavored yogurt, pasta sauce, salad dressing, and granola bars, to name a few. You think you're making a healthy choice, but you're ingesting a hidden sugar bomb. In 2012 the Centers for Disease Control and Prevention reported that children consumed from 282 calories (girls) to 362 calories (boys) of added sugars per day. Savvy shoppers know to avoid the obvious ones like sugar, high fructose corn syrup, and even agave nectar. But there are numerous other hidden sweeteners with more cloaked names such as cane crystals, maltodextrin, evaporated cane juice, and sorghum syrup. That's why it's so important to read the ingredient list on foods—especially those that come in jars, packages, and boxes—to avoid those containing too many added sugars.

The new 2015–2020 *Dietary Guidelines for Americans* recommends consuming 10 percent or less of your total calories from added sugars. That's all well and good, but I am sure you are wondering how in the world you're supposed to figure that out. Well, by mid-2018 "Added Sugars" will actually be listed under the "Carbohydrate" section on the Nutrition Facts Panel of foods, making it much easier to spot. Until then, and even after, you should examine the ingredient list—each of which is listed in order of how much of it is in the product. For example, if there are ten ingredients in a box of pita chips and the tenth ingredient is maltodextrin or corn syrup (aka sugar), then you know there is likely not as much sugar in that product. However, if it is the first or second ingredient on the list, then that is probably a food with a high added sugar content and you should find an alternative to dip in your hummus. Plus, looking for a smaller number of ingredients all the way around usually means the food item is less processed and likely does not have as many additives. I'm not asking you to bust out a calculator in the cereal aisle, but being aware can help you make better food choices.

LOW-CALORIE SWEETENERS

The steady drumbeat over the years to eat less sugar is really what has made the low-calorie (artificial) sweetener category so popular. Aspartame, saccharin, sucralose, sugar alcohols, and more "natural" choices such as stevia and monk fruit are among a larger list able to sweeten foods without adding calories. Note that sugar alcohols—made popular in the "no-carb" era—are not calorie-free and can actually yield almost as many calories as glucose (sugar) per gram. Many people think they are eating sugar-free with these ingredients when really they might just be eating a tiny bit less.

While there is some debate over the long-term effects of these artificial sweeteners, there is no definitive proof that frequent consumption poses health risks for healthy individuals, and the Food and Drug Administration (FDA) has deemed them safe to consume. If anyone tells you they heard they cause cancer, tell them the National Cancer Institute disagrees. There's also some theory that low-calorie sweeteners impair the body's ability to receive an adequate sugar "fix," since it's getting something sweet but with no calories to show for it. So the body's natural intuition about its caloric needs is thrown out of whack, leading to overeating. Still, a 2014 meta-analysis of randomized controlled trials published in the *American Journal of Clinical Nutrition* concluded that substituting low-calorie sweeteners for sugar resulted in modest loss in body weight, body mass index (BMI), and waist circumference. In other words, if you're trying to cut pounds, low-calorie sweeteners are probably a better conduit than regular sugar and have been shown to be a successful tool in weight-loss efforts.

But what I'd like to impress upon you is that neither option should be abused. Consuming ridiculously large amounts of any sweetener—real or artificial—should not be a part of a healthy lifestyle. If you like a Splenda in your morning coffee, or go for the occasional ice cream indulgence—it's one of my favorites—that's not going to derail your fitness goals or cause health consequences. However, if you need everything you eat to have an overly sweet taste—your peanut butter needs to be honey roasted, your cereal needs frosting—you likely don't have a healthy relationship with food. That has to change. Start looking at nutrition labels and ingredients lists to spot unnecessary added sugars. Use tablespoons to measure out portion sizes of garnishes and toppings—not squeezes—and become aware of how much sweetness you might be putting in food or in a recipe. Swap in alternatives like mustard, hot sauce, and rubs to add low-calorie flavoring to food instead of creamy, sugary dressings and marinades. Learn to taste food that is less sweet and appreciate the flavor of whole foods. It may not be overnight, but with some discipline and simple food substitutions you'll be able to lessen the amount of sweetness in your diet.

GLUTEN-FREE

If you ask most people what "gluten-free" means they generally don't know, but those adhering to the lifestyle will be absolutely certain it's a "healthier" choice. For those unfamiliar with the details of this spreading diet trend, indulge me in a brief introduction. Gluten is the protein in wheat and thus in all whole-wheat products like spelt, kamut, farro, and durum, plus products like bulgur, semolina, barley, rye, and triticale. Oats don't naturally contain gluten but are typically made in facilities that produce wheat products, which is why some oat products can't make the claim of being completely gluten-free.

As those sound like perfectly good whole-grain complex carbohydrates, why would anyone choose to cut gluten out of their diets?

The only legitimate reason is a medical one. A small percentage of the population—approximately 1 percent—has something called *celiac disease*. These people are actually allergic to gluten. If they consume it, they get very sick with gastrointestinal distress such as cramping, bloating, sharp pains, and gas, and, more important, they will malabsorb both macro- and micronutrients. This can lead to a host of health issues and deficiencies. Thus they have to choose gluten-free grains like corn, millet, rice, sorghum, amaranth, buckwheat, quinoa, and gluten-free oats.

They can also choose breads, crackers, and the like made with potato and sweet potato flour. As gluten is commonly used in many sauces and spreads, those who need to absolutely avoid it have to be vigilant when they eat. People with celiac disease tend to look for high-fiber versions of these products, since it's easy to miss out on fiber when whole wheat and associated products are eliminated.

So for perfectly legitimate health reasons, a tiny fraction of people need to banish gluten. Why then does another 30 percent or more of the population choose gluten-free foods? Another small percentage—less than 8 percent—has non-celiac gluten sensitivity (NCGS). This means they experience many of the same symptoms of those with celiac disease when they consume gluten. However, they may or may not malabsorb nutrients.

But the rest of the population eating gluten-free have likely gotten caught up in "popular science," generally the result of the media jumping on a nutrient or product and vilifying it—as discussed earlier, a fate suffered by many carbohydrates. People think they are eating healthy as they have been convinced that gluten is harmful, when really the opposite is true. Not only are whole wheat and gluten-containing grains rich in fiber, they are also high in B vitamins, iron, and folic acid. When people cut out gluten from their diet, they're missing an opportunity to consume these valuable nutrients.

Bottom line: unless you have celiac disease or NCGS, there's absolutely no reason to avoid these high-fiber foods. If you are asking yourself, "I wonder if I have this disease or sensitivity?," statistically speaking, the answer is likely no. And trust me, you would know if you did—your gastrointestinal tract would be hollering at you every time you ate even a few bites of gluten. Don't fall for the hype. Again, it's likely not whole-grain foods bulging people's waistlines; it's processed products laden with added sugar consumed in excess that creates a surplus of calories over the course of the day. So fear not. Go forth and eat nutrient-rich whole grains.

Eating the right amount of carbohydrates at meals can be tricky. An easy shortcut to striking a healthful balance is to partition your plate into three sections. I didn't invent this practice, and percentages can vary, but it's quite effective, especially if you're not a fan of calorie counting. At mealtime—this applies more to lunch and dinner than breakfast—cover 50 percent of your plate with fibrous vegetables. Stack them high. Eat them raw, roasted, or grilled. Don't even worry how much is there. As long as you don't cover them with cheese, heavy sauces, or lots of oil, it will be a nutrient powerhouse that will help eliminate fat rather than put it on.

Next, save another 25 percent of the plate for your protein. We'll get to the various sources in the next chapter, but lean meats and fish are always a good choice. Whenever possible, opt for seasonings and rubs over marinades to keep the calorie count in check.

The final 25 percent goes to a complex carbohydrate or starchy vegetable—sweet potato, corn, brown rice, couscous, and so on. By limiting the space allotted to these higher-calorie carbs, you can still draw their health benefits—and the psychological comfort of enjoying such pleasurable foods—without overindulging. Note that as your exercise training and minutes ramp up, it can be appropriate to divide your plate into thirds, especially if you are feeling tired or lethargic throughout the day. Again, carbohydrate need is heavily based on activity level, so the more you move, the more you are able to consume.

CHAPTER 8

BUILDING (ENGINE) BLOCKS

Let food be thy medicine and medicine be thy food.

When you lift weights or apply some form of external load to the body, it causes damage and breaks down the targeted muscle. For instance, pump out several sets of dumbbell curls and you attack the biceps, causing microtears in the muscle. When you leave the gym and rest, the body repairs the biceps, causing it to adapt, grow, and fill out your shirtsleeve. The nutritive element to the equation is dietary protein. If our sports-car bodies incur dings and dents from exercise, protein consumption is how we restore and bolster them so they get stronger and better than ever.

As much as carbohydrates have been vilified lately, high-protein diets have been deified. Proteins not only are vital for active people and play a variety of roles in the body, they also take longer to digest than carbs while containing the same 4 calories per gram. That's why two whole large eggs—approximately 150 calories from protein and fat—satisfy hunger better than two pieces of toast—150 to 180 calories, mostly from carbs. But when the two are combined at breakfast, it helps stabilize blood sugar. This keeps a consistent, steady flow of energy to the body, rather than a quick high followed by a crash. So protein gets you full faster and keeps you satisfied longer, and this is why it's included in all meals and snacks in our sample meal plans.

There are lots of opinions on how much protein sedentary versus active people should consume on a daily basis. Many tout protein as the savior for all weight-loss programs. It seems you can't eat enough of it, and it should be the first thing you reach for when you're hungry. But, as with any nutrient, you can still get plenty tubby by making every burger a double. Some of you might be familiar with the Recommended Dietary Allowance (RDA), which recommends 0.8 gram protein per kilogram of body weight for "generally healthy" sedentary people to maintain normal daily function and prevent nutrient deficiency.

HOW DO YOU KNOW WHAT YOU WEIGH IN KILOGRAMS?

Take your weight in pounds, divide it by 2.2, and there is your answer. So a 200-pound man weighs 91 kilograms. Under the RDA, if this 200-pound man is sedentary, he would need approximately 73 grams of protein (0.8 gram per kilogram of body weight) a day to maintain health. If you're trying to lose weight, including more protein in a diet helps with satiety, stokes the body's metabolism, and helps maintain muscle mass despite being in a caloric deficit. And people on an exercise program like mine need more protein to preserve and build lean body mass. Plus as you age, muscle and metabolic rate naturally decline, so consuming more protein can help maintain the muscle mass you have and fight off sarcopenia (decreased muscle mass).

For those reasons, I tend to side with eating a little too much protein, rather than too little. But you still must be reasoned in your intake. What's the proper amount? Trying to decipher that from the so-called diet experts populating the media only causes more confusion. Some recommend that athletes and people involved in serious training programs—like this one—need massive loads of protein to maintain and build muscle; some say that too much protein is bad for the kidneys; and some claim it can even cause cancer. With so much conflicting information and opinions, it's important to know what science actually says. So my policy is to seek a healthy balance, not perfection, and use my sports dietitian's guidelines for myself and when talking nutrition with my clients. Here's a simple formula you can use to determine how much protein you should be consuming per day:

Activity Level	Recommended Protein Needs
Sedentary (no exercise)	0.8 gm/kg body weight
Moderately active (a few days a week)	1.0 gm/kg body weight
Endurance athletes (runners, cyclists, swimmers)	1.2 to 1.4 gm/kg body weight
Weight loss (with activity included)	1.5 gm/kg body weight
Strength athletes	1.6 to 1.7 gm/kg body weight
Heavy-strength-training athletes	1.7 to 2.0 gm/kg body weight

My weight: _____ lbs. divided by 2.2 = _____ kg

My weight _____ kg multiplied by the amount of protein required for my activity level _____ gm/kg = _____ gm of protein per day for ME

Basically, if you have a clean protein source at each meal, and a smaller one when snacking, you should be close to what you need without obsessing over the total. However, learning the appropriate amounts of protein for your activity level and body size will make it easier not to regularly over- or underconsume what you need. So bust out your calculator to get an idea of your daily requirement; then use these easy real-life items to help calculate protein amounts when you are eating at home or out in a restaurant:

PROTEIN-COUNTING CHART

Food	Grams of Protein	Portion Size Example
3 oz. lean meat, chicken, turkey, pork, tofu	21 to 24 grams	Deck of cards or the palm of a woman's hand
3 oz. fish	18 to 22 grams	Checkbook
1 cup yogurt	8 to 12 grams	Baseball
1 oz. cheese	7 to 10 grams	Tube of lip gloss
2 Tbsp. peanut butter	8 grams	Golf ball

PROTEIN SOURCES

Amino acids are the building blocks of protein, and they are responsible for fixing and repairing what training has damaged in the body. There are technically twenty-two (commonly thought of as twenty) amino acids that work to keep the body in stellar condition, nine of them being essential—meaning they cannot be made in the body and must be consumed from food. The rest of them are found in food but can also be made in the body from other amino acids, thus making them nonessential. Animal foods such as chicken, beef, pork, turkey, fish, dairy, and eggs contain all nine essential amino acids, making them complete proteins; plant foods like beans, legumes, nuts and nut butters, seeds, and whole grains do not contain all nine essentials, making them incomplete proteins. Soy is the outlier, as it is a plant food with all nine essential amino acids. Thus, soy foods like soy milk/yogurt, tempeh, tofu, and edamame are considered complete proteins along with quinoa, a high-protein grain. So if you follow a plant-based diet you need to get a variety of plant proteins on the menu to ensure that you're getting enough protein and all the essential amino acids to keep your sports-car body in pristine shape.

Other ways to do that include getting in *complementary proteins*—two foods that together give you all nine essential amino acids. Keep in mind you do not have to do this at each meal, but combinations like black beans and brown rice, bean salad with corn and couscous, peanut butter on whole-wheat bread, or even trail mix with nuts, seeds, and toasted oats can help increase the protein in your day, ensuring that you are getting everything you need.

As with most food, there are high- and low-quality protein options to choose from. Ideally you want to choose lean protein—lean meaning low in fat. Animal foods naturally have fat; there is skin on chicken, gristle on meat, and fat in dairy. To get the protein without all the added fat, you have to consciously make lean decisions:

1. Take the skin off your chicken or turkey, or opt for skinless breast meat
2. Buy lean cuts of red meat and cut off visible fat
3. Choose low-fat or fat-free dairy
4. Bake, grill, and pan-sear instead of frying
5. Go fish—it's naturally lean

Plant foods, on the other hand, are naturally lean, having zero animal fat. If you are eating a plant-based diet, choosing high-protein plant foods like beans, nuts, seeds, and whole grains, as mentioned earlier, is essential. Just be careful to monitor your intake. Foods like beans and whole grains are carb-rich, and nuts and seeds are high in fat, which results in higher calories. If you eat large quantities to meet your protein demands, you must be mindful that doing so doesn't result in your exceeding your daily caloric limit.

PROTEIN SUPPLEMENTS

The supplement industry is a multibillion-dollar behemoth. Health and nutrition stores are the new Starbucks. You can't walk through a mall without coming across a GNC or Vitamin Shoppe, and even supermarkets are now devoting aisles to these products. The multitude of drinks, powders, bars, and pills designed to help people lose weight, build muscle, and crush their workouts appears endless. The offers many of these products make can be quite seductive—who doesn't want to become ripped and muscular by simply swallowing a pill?—and the reason people are so willing to part with their cash to purchase them.

However, an important thing to keep in mind is that the supplement industry is also largely unregulated. This means that a lot of these products don't contain the levels they purport to have, masking their makeup with dubious "proprietary blends" or using sub-standard ingredients. In other words, it's junk. And oftentimes, rather expensive junk. That doesn't mean there aren't quality supplements on the market. But you need to do your own research and choose third-party-tested supplements—I don't recommend trusting the store clerk pushing a particular brand at a nutrition store.

Which is why at this point in my life I don't take any supplements. I don't have any-thing against the practice. I used to take creatine—a popular mass-builder—to keep my weight up when I played in the NFL. Even now if I'm dragging I'll take a preworkout energy drink to get my blood pumping before hitting the gym. But it's not something I do on a regular basis. I believe if you're smart and dedicated to eating the right foods, you'll get all the nutrition you need at mealtime.

That said, I appreciate the value that some people put on protein supplements. You'd have to be living under a rock in the fitness world not to have noticed the prevalence of whey protein in everything from bars and powders to pancakes and bagels. Not bad for the castoff of curdled milk. Many studies claim that having a postworkout whey protein shake can enhance lean muscle mass and aid in recovery. Again, I don't subscribe, but if you find it helps and it's a good opportunity to meet your protein requirements, I'm not one to argue. Sports dietitians recommend high-quality protein (whey is a milk protein and thus considered high-quality with all the essential amino acids) after a workout to help muscles repair and rebuild. Many choose protein shakes out of convenience to get protein in as quickly as possible, so if that is you, then I can see where a smoothie made with whey protein, fruit, and water, or a ready-to-drink shake, might be a good option. The sample daily meal plans in this book even offer suggestions for protein bars to have as snacks to meet the need for convenience. And for vegans and vegetarians who find it difficult to get enough protein through whole foods, options like pea, hemp, and brown rice protein powders can help fill in the gaps.

But I think you've got to earn the right to use it. Work hard in the gym, follow a clean and healthy diet, and then you can use supplements like protein powders to augment your training, or as a quick option when you are in a hurry. Some people eat poorly and exercise sporadically but think they're making up for it by drinking a pricey "superfood" shake. That won't help. Never forget, it's called a supplement—not a substitute. If your workouts are lacking and you've got a junk-filled diet, there's nothing you can buy in a bottle that will save you. That money would be better spent discovering the superfoods in the produce aisle.

CHAPTER 9
GREASE THE WHEELS

Without deviation, progress is not possible. —**Frank Zappa**

It undoubtedly has something to do with the name, but there's a common misconception that eating fat—the third member of the holy trinity of macronutrients—makes you fat. Ill-informed dieters stock up on "fat-free" and "light" foods, believing them to be healthier choices. However, what these foods may lack in fats, they often lack in taste. To compensate, they're regularly loaded with sugar, unhealthy chemicals (or additives), and flavor substitutes that can end up being more damaging to the body than natural fats. And since these Frankenfoods tend to be less satisfying, people tend to eat more of them, which ultimately can lead to extra, unneeded calories.

Eliminating fats won't prevent someone from being overweight—monitoring calories will. (Sound familiar?) Perhaps one of the more illuminating and humorous examples of this is the now-famous Twinkie Diet. A professor of nutrition at Kansas State University lost 27 pounds over 10 weeks on a diet primarily composed of Twinkies and other junk foods such as Oreos and Doritos. Along with some multivitamins, he basically subsisted on sugar and fat. His dentist must have been horrified. He limited himself to 1,800 calories a day, about 800 less than a man of his size would require to maintain his body weight. Here's the even crazier part: in the process he dropped his body fat, lowered his triglycerides by 39 percent, reduced his LDL or "bad" cholesterol by 20 percent, and raised his HDL or "good" cholesterol by the same percentage. That's right, he ate a vending-machine diet and his health appears to have benefited from it.

Now, as tasty as it might be, in no way would I advocate a meal plan consisting of snack cakes and processed junk. Besides being unsustainable for the long term, it doesn't provide enough nutrients or protein for the body, especially for a person involved in regular physical activity. Not to mention it would be virtually impossible to get your kids to eat their veggies. But it does show that dieting isn't as simple as vilifying a particular food group.

However, while a calorie might be a calorie in weight loss, nutrient-wise, calories can differ greatly. For instance, a tablespoon of mayonnaise has 90 calories and 10 grams of fat, while a tablespoon of peanut butter has a similar 95 calories and 8 grams of fat. Both are high in fat, but peanut butter's fat is unsaturated while mayonnaise's is saturated, not to mention that peanut butter is pumped with iron, protein, and other essential nutrients, making it a smart food choice. Mayo? Not so much. Beyond sticking to a calorie range that maintains a healthy body weight, you want those calories to be impactful—high in nutrients and low in junk.

As a side note, most doctors will tell you that a decent amount of weight loss, even 10 percent of total body weight, will typically improve blood cholesterol, triglyceride, and blood pressure numbers. That's what happened with the professor subscribing to the Twinkie Diet. However, the key is keeping the weight off long-term to maintain those numbers, and that can be accomplished only with a healthy, sustainable eating pattern and regular exercise.

GET TO KNOW YOUR FAT

Heart Health Numbers	Optimal Range	Ways to Improve
Total cholesterol	Less than 200 mg/dL	Decrease saturated and trans fat intake Increase soluble-fiber intake Lose weight Exercise
LDL (bad) cholesterol	Less than 100 mg/dL	Decrease saturated and trans fat intake Increase soluble-fiber intake Lose weight Exercise
HDL (good) cholesterol	Men: Greater than 40 mg/dL Women: Greater than 50 mg/dL	Increase unsaturated fat intake, specifically omega-3 fatty acids Exercise
Triglycerides	Less than 150 mg/dL	Decrease saturated and trans fat intake Increase unsaturated fat intake, specifically omega-3 fatty acids Decrease processed-carbohydrate intake Lose weight Exercise
Blood pressure	Less than 120/80 mmHg	Lose weight Exercise Decrease salt intake

The skinny on fat is that it is essential to the diet just like carbohydrate and protein. But eat too much of it and it will indeed live up to its name. Think of dietary fat to your body like oil that lubricates a car's engine—it's necessary for it to function properly, but needed in smaller amounts when compared to gas. Fat yields 9 calories per gram versus the 4 calories per gram from carbohydrate and protein. So spreading fat intake judiciously throughout a meal plan is key. Twenty almonds with fruit can make a great snack; 65 almonds can turn into a caloric avalanche.

But fat doesn't just provide calories, it plays a variety of roles in the body. It helps transport and store the fat-soluble vitamins A, D, E, and K and helps in hormone production, protecting internal organs, maintaining healthy skin, and adding to meal satiety. Unlike a quick hit of sugar, fat helps you feel like you ate something. Think of the last time you had pizza—you likely inhaled a few slices and didn't think about food for several hours. Between the oil, cheese, and various meat toppings, there can be a day's worth of fat on a single slice of pizza. I don't want you to eat pizza every night, but in our meal plans, you will see foods like avocado and seeds added to a salad, or hummus to a sandwich wrap to help give you that satisfied feeling.

So while many diets will tell you to treat fat like an irritating relative—experienced as infrequently as possible—it should be an integral part of any effective eating plan. In fact, the low-fat guidelines outlined in the *Dietary Goals for the United States* were first published by the government in 1977 and since that point obesity rates have ballooned. Obviously we can't blame fat for the obesity epidemic. The problem likely lies in portion sizes of healthy and processed food, not to mention added sugars and fats that fill the ingredient lists of many packaged foods. Actually, the current 2015–2020 *Dietary Guidelines for Americans* welcomes fat as part of a healthy diet. The key is choosing more of the "good" fats and avoiding/limiting the "bad" fats that don't have the same health benefits. What are good and bad fats? Well, I'm glad you asked, because it needs to be front and center when you are making food decisions.

FAT BURNERS

Fatty Food Choice	Exercise Needed to Burn It Off
Big Mac (490 calories)	3 hours, 8 minutes of Rollerblading
16 oz. Frappuccino (500 calories)	2 hours, 10 minutes of Pilates
Slice of pizza (285 calories)	1,425 sit-ups
Cheesecake (1,000 calories)	1,408 burpees
Chocolate croissant (300 calories)	Walk dog for 2 hours
Large French fries (600 calories)	1.5 hours of swimming
Glazed doughnut (190 calories)	53 minutes of lunges
Chocolate bar (240 calories)	21 minutes of jumping rope
Cinnabon (730 calories)	1 hour, 20 minutes of cycling at 12.5 mph

GOOD FATS

Just like carbs and proteins, there are also different grades of fat that influence its nutritional impact. Unsaturated fats—mono and poly—are categorized as good fats. Monounsaturated fats are plant-based fats that are liquid at room temperature, such as olive, peanut, and sunflower oil. Avocados, nuts, and seeds also contain fatty acids that can help lower bad (LDL) cholesterol and triglyceride levels while contributing to improving good cholesterol levels (HDL). If you want good blood flow and a healthy ticker, stick with these fats.

MONOUNSATURATED FATS LIST

Olive oil

Sunflower oil

Cashews

Hazelnuts

Macadamia nuts

Almonds

Pistachios

Sesame seeds

Nut butters

Halibut

Mackerel

Avocados

Olives

Polyunsaturated fat provides the two essential fatty acids that the body cannot make: omega-3 and omega-6 fatty acids, or linolenic and linoleic acids. While the Western diet is high in omega-6 fatty acids (plant-based), most Americans do not consume enough omega-3 fatty acids, which is a shame as these polyunsaturated fats help decrease inflammation at the cellular level. Oils rich in these fats can also increase the amount of vitamin E, an antioxidant that helps combat free radicals in the body and that many Americans also need in greater abundance. (This is why many turn to supplements to increase their omega-3 and vitamin E intake.) So eat your salmon. Ideally you want about 10 percent of your total calories to come from monounsaturated fat and 10 percent from polyunsaturated.

POLYUNSATURATED FATS LIST

Canola oil

Soybeans and soybean oil

Walnuts

Chia seeds

Flaxseeds

Salmon

Tuna

Sardines

Mackerel

Egg yolk

"BAD" FATS

Saturated and trans fats—the so-called bad fats—can contribute to inflammation in the body and raise blood levels of cholesterol when consumed in excess. Hence, the derogatory label. Saturated fats come from animal foods and are primarily found in meat; full-fat dairy products; white, thick, and creamy foods; and baked goods. Recent research has lessened the guilt of eating saturated fat, supporting the idea that they can make up a small percentage of fat intake. The American Heart Association recommends that 10 percent or less of total calories come from this type of fat. However, just as calories can pack a different nutrient punch, small amounts of saturated fat from sautéing veggies in a little coconut oil, having full-fat milk at breakfast, or a hard-boiled egg for a snack can boost nutrients and protein. In other words, in moderation the pros outweigh the cons. Slathering fried chicken in gravy, dipping fish sticks in tartar sauce, and dousing noodles with creamy Alfredo sauce, while delicious to some, doesn't provide quite the same nutrient bang for your buck.

SATURATED FATS LIST

Whole-fat dairy foods

Butter

Gristled and marbled beef

Skin-on chicken

Palm oil

Palm kernel oil

Coconut oil

White, thick, and creamy foods like ranch and Caesar salad dressings,
mayonnaise, Alfredo sauce, tartar sauce, gravy, whipped cream, and
cream cheese

Trans fats are basically off-limits because they are typically artificially formed instead of naturally occurring—for example, hydrogen is added to vegetable oils to make them more solid—thus making them more dangerous in the body. You might recognize trans fat in an ingredient list as "hydrogenated or partially hydrogenated"—but it might as well be labeled "slow-acting poison"—and its presence improves the flavoring, texture, and shelf life of packaged foods. Eating trans fats has been shown to raise bad (LDL) cholesterol while lowering good (HDL) cholesterol and increasing the risk of heart disease and stroke. High consumption has also been linked to developing type 2 diabetes. There are no nutrient or health benefits of any kind from consuming trans fat.

Beginning in 2006, trans fats were required to be listed on the Nutrition Facts Panel to help consumers better identify them in products. At that point many manufacturers and even fast-food chains began using different oils to help decrease and ultimately remove trans fat from foods. In 2013, the FDA determined that partially hydrogenated oils are no longer generally recognized as safe in human food, and in 2015 it mandated that manufacturers totally remove trans fat from their foods within three years—thanks for the memories. Not to belabor the obvious, but avoid trans fats whenever possible.

TRANS FATS LIST

Fried fast foods

Margarine

Shortening (like Crisco)

Packaged cookies and cakes

Processed foods containing partially hydrogenated oil

Doughnuts and many pastry-type foods

Microwave popcorn

FAT CHANCES

Because fat provides the body with more calories per bite, sprinkling it throughout the day at meals and snacks is the best way to fit it in without adding jiggle to your middle. Unlike vegetables, you're not consciously looking to load up on fatty foods. Think of a garnish on a plate at a restaurant and now picture fitting fat into your meals in that manner:

- Sprinkle nuts on your oatmeal at breakfast
- Dip your apple in peanut butter as a midmorning snack
- Add avocado to your wrap at lunch
- Decorate your pita chips with hummus in the afternoon
- Roast your veggies in olive oil and serve them with salmon and sweet potato for dinner

Remember, the great thing about fat, besides being nutrient-rich, is that it helps you feel satisfied after a meal. Instead of feeling like you need another bite of something, fat helps you appreciate the savoriness of a meal. Just remember to keep consumption under control. Ideally you want to keep fat to 20 to 35 percent of your total calorie intake. If you consistently go higher than that, your jeans size will follow suit.

FAT SWAPS

High-Fat Food	Healthy Swap
Alfredo sauce	Marinara sauce
Mayonnaise	Mustard
Cream cheese	Peanut butter
Creamy salad dressing	Balsamic vinaigrette
Tartar sauce	Ketchup
Butter/margarine	Yogurt-based butter
French fries	Roasted sweet potato wedges
Biscuit	English muffin
Doughnut or pastry	Whole-wheat toast
Fried chicken	Grilled or pan-seared chicken

CHAPTER 10

COOLANTS

Thousands have lived without love, not one without water.

—W. H. Auden

Hydration and adequate fluid consumption isn't a sexy topic, but it's a largely over-looked component of proper nutrition. Look at it this way: your body can survive much longer without food than it can without water. Watch any survival movie like *127 Hours* or *Unbroken* and the heroes are desperate for water, not steak. Depending on age, the human body is composed of 60 to 80 percent water, making it essential that you're hydrating throughout the day, every single day. The general guideline is to consume half your body weight (in pounds) in ounces of fluid per day. So if you weigh 180 pounds, you need to drink 90 ounces of fluids every day. Exercise will increase this intake, requiring an additional 5 to 10 ounces for every 20 minutes of consistent activity.

Falling short of your fluid requirements is easier and more troublesome than you think. In fact, most people are walking around dehydrated on a daily basis. How do you know if you are hydrated? While it may not be the most elegant exam, the easiest way to tell is to actually look at the color of your urine. Yup, pee is the best test—pale yellow to clear is generally deemed hydrated; the color of apple juice and darker usu-ally means dehydrated. You are more likely to be dehydrated when you wake up in the morning, when it is really hot and humid outside, and/or if you work out twice a day. These are times when you may need to drink more than what is customary for you. Keep in mind: even mild dehydration can cause dizziness, muscle cramps, and fatigue.

Where most people get tripped up is in the types of fluids they are putting in their bodies. The biggest pitfall is not paying enough attention to the sugar content—and thus calories—in certain drinks. Beverages such as sodas, sweetened teas, fruit juices, lemonade, smoothies, fancy coffee beverages, sports drinks when not exercising, and alcohol can add up to tons of sugar calories over the course of the day. Yes, you need carbohydrate, but the sugar found in these beverages is mostly just the added varieties. They provide zero feelings of fullness, so you end up drinking hundreds of calories on top of your regular meals. And just because you drink your calories doesn't mean they count any less than those consumed through solid foods. So the goal is to stay hydrated without breaking your calorie budget.

WATER

The pound-for-pound undisputed champ in the hydration department remains water. Your body is about 60 percent water—your blood is 92 percent—and it functions much better when filled to capacity. Adequate water consumption aids with digestion and blood circulation, keeps muscles firing, and has even been shown to lower the risk of bladder cancer and kidney stones. Oh yeah, and it packs a whopping zero calories. All that from three atoms.

The problem is that drinking plain water can be plain boring. Some people simply can't get around the absence of taste, not to mention that many people don't "feel" thirsty over the course of the day when they're not working out. So when they do drink—a sports drink during exercise, a soda with a snack—they'd rather it be something that goes down easily and that they enjoy. I find that drinking water to wash down food with meals can be an easy way to reach your hydration quota. Drink a 16-ounce bottle of water with each meal or snack—our meal plan recommends 5 to 6 bottles per day—and you'll be up to around 96 ounces. If you enjoy carbonated drinks, naturally flavored seltzers have zero calories and can be more pleasurable and easier to drink than plain water. Don't forget, fruits and vegetables have high concentrations of water too, so if you're eating several servings a day you'll be adding to your hydration levels.

One important thing to note is that just because water is good for you doesn't mean you have to attach a gallon jug to your hip and chug it down at the top of every hour. In fact, don't do that. If you can see a theme with the nutrition information in this book, it's that just because a little is good doesn't mean a lot is better. Too much water can actually be detrimental. Drinking excessive amounts of it can lead to over-hydration, which can throw off the balance between water and sodium in your blood. So drink plenty of water, but don't overflow in it.

COFFEE AND TEA

No longer just for breakfast, coffee and tea drinks are now all-day companions. Numerous potential health benefits are linked to this duo: fat loss, increased essential nutrients and antioxidants, improved mood, increased energy levels, and even low-ered risk of certain diseases. After all, tea leaves and coffee beans come from plants, which are full of righteous stuff for the body. There was a belief that consuming coffee and other caffeinated beverages—certain teas have little to no caffeine—leads to dehydration. But that myth has since been debunked—these drinks can have a diuretic effect, but it doesn't impact hydration levels over a twenty-four-hour period. So any tea or coffee you drink throughout the day adds to your hydration total. However, be mindful of how much caffeine you're consuming—it's recommended not to exceed 500 milligrams per day—as excessive amounts can lead to trouble sleeping and irritability, and potentially have a dehydrating effect. Not to mention it can make you just plain wired. Also, many people are caffeine sensitive and a small amount can have a major impact on your central nervous system.

The other caveat with these drinks is that while they are low calorie when simply combined with boiling water, they become quite the opposite when accompanied by frothy milk or cream, drizzled with sugary toppings, and basically turned into a dessert. Lots of bottled teas also come loaded with added sugars. I'd be lying if I said I didn't enjoy sweet tea with my meals, but drinking glasses of it with dinner is like having a side of gummy bears. Consuming just a couple of these drinks can add several hundred calories to a daily total without much nutritional benefit. Plus, in the case of the designer coffee drinks, you'll be riding the wave of sugar and caffeine energy spikes and crashes. Skip the whipped cream and caramel, and get your java fix as close to naked as possible.

SODA

For the most part, regular soda is nothing more than liquid candy. Yes, drinking a lot of it can keep you hydrated. However, all the added sugars and unwanted calories are way too destructive to your overall health—bad for the waistline and teeth and full of questionable additives. Some varieties are lower in sugar and may even try to sell themselves as a "healthy" soda, but it's still something that should be consumed as more of an occasional treat.

Which is why so many people rely on diet soda. I'm sure you know someone who has a diet soda addiction. These drinks generally save you the 140+ calories of regular soda (and that's just for a 12-ounce can) by relying on artificial or low-calorie sweeteners for taste. The FDA deems these sweeteners safe, as mentioned in Chapter 7, but again, you don't want to overdo it. Diet soda can be a way to decrease caloric intake if you enjoy flavor in your beverage. Also, it often is a great tool in weight loss if you are replacing a regular soda's calories with zero calories from diet soda.

Remember, though, that low-calorie sweeteners are typically 200 to 600 times sweeter than actual sucrose or table sugar. The potent sweet taste, with extended use, can desensitize you to naturally sweet foods. In other words, if it's not cotton-candy-level sweet, you won't like it. Be aware, too, that low-calorie sweeteners don't register with the body like sugar does. So if you are craving something sweet and drink a diet soda, or anything artificially sweetened, you may not satisfy that craving. This leaves many people searching for something else sweet, then blaming diet soda for weight gain. Think about it: if you drink a 12-ounce can of diet soda to satisfy your sweet tooth, but then follow it 30 minutes later with a grande Frappuccino because you still want something sugary, then you didn't replace the calories in a regular soda. You might have actually consumed more sugar with the frothy drink.

I'm not saying diet soda is full of nutrients, or that a soda here and there will make you gain 10 pounds. Drinking a reasonable amount of diet soda—a can or two per day—is probably not a problem for most people. Having a regular soda with your family on pizza night won't kill you either. But neither option possesses much nutritional value, and you're better off replacing it whenever possible with water.

FRUIT JUICES AND SMOOTHIES

Pomegranate, mangosteen, guava—you name the fruit and it now comes juiced in a bottle. While many fruits do have health benefits such as vitamins and antioxidants, they're also often loaded with calories because fruit is made of fructose, which is sugar. In fact, some juice varieties pack more sugar than a can of soda. But because fruit is natural and nutrient-rich, some people give it a pass, especially parents looking to get their kids to drink something. The truth is you're always better off eating an actual piece of fruit; the flesh contains the fiber and many of the nutrients. Plus, it's a better use of calories: a typical orange is about 60 calories, while an 8-ounce glass of orange juice is around 140 calories and not nearly as satisfying.

Vegetable juice is lower in calories than pure fruit juices but suffers from the missing nutritional benefits of roughage (fiber). It also takes a lot of vegetables to create the juice, but since it's juice it provides no fullness to the stomach. And straight veggie juice can also taste a little too earthy, which is why fruit juice is often added to improve the sweetness. So unless you have a strong aversion to fruits and vegetables and can reap only a few of their benefits in liquid form, you're much better off eating the whole version.

If you do want to juice, the best way is to create a base with vegetables and then add two servings of fruit (see Chapter 7 for serving sizes). This allows you to have a fairly sweet, nutrient-packed juice for way fewer calories than fruit alone. Another option is to blend the whole fruit or vegetable. Many high-powered, fancy blenders on the market have this capability and allow you to get the nutrients and fiber, which can aid in satiety.

A smoothie is a more filling option that can constitute a snack or even an entire meal. You can go small with something as simple as Greek yogurt, some milk, and a handful of berries; or you can dress it up into a more elaborate concoction with scoops of protein powder, milk, peanut butter, fruits, and sweetener. The former tops off at about 150 calories, and the latter will billow to over 500 calories. I have seen people order smoothies with a meal when really the smoothie should *be* the meal. Don't get tricked by the lure of "health" by the brightly lit, catchy-sounding smoothie store. Some smoothies are worthwhile, but they're not always the best option. Many are loaded with added sugar and lack protein. A few smoothie tips:

- Get a "skinny." Most smoothie places add turbinado, a fancy type of sugar, to all of their smoothies. "Skinny" usually means the sugar in it came only from fruit or fruit juice.
- Check the protein. When thinking smoothies, most people think protein, but amazingly enough many of these thick drinks have less than 5 grams. If you're drinking a smoothie as a meal replacement, look for one with at least 20 to 30 grams of protein. Choosing a flavor made with milk or yogurt will help boost the protein content.
- Get a small. Again, sugar calories coming from fruit can add up quickly. Smoothies can run in the 500-to-700-calorie range with more than 100 grams of carbohydrate. By ordering a small size, you naturally will get less of it. If you are getting a smoothie as a snack, consider a kiddie size and (again) make sure it has protein.

Smoothies and postworkout shakes are popular after exercise, but you still have to include them in your daily caloric budget. Some people drink a postworkout smoothie so dense that they replace more calories than they burned off. Again, liquid calories add up quickly, even if they're filled with nutrients. If you're a regular smoothie drinker, take a few minutes and plug all your ingredients into a fitness/nutrition app to see how many calories it has; or, if you swing by your gym café after your morning workout, go online and look up the nutritional content of your favorite bottled smoothie. Awareness is key and can help keep you from sabotaging yourself when you thought you were actually doing right by your body.

ENERGY AND SPORTS DRINKS

Having Gatorade or a similar type of sports drink during a workout or while playing a sport can help maintain performance during the activity. While many complain about the sugar content, the quick hit of sugar, along with some electrolytes, can keep the body hydrated and energized. This is especially true for long workouts. The rule of thumb is that if you are working out for less than 60 to 90 minutes, you are likely fine with just water at regular intervals. Activity lasting 90 minutes or more requires consistent carbohydrate intake to maintain energy levels. For most of us hitting the gym, water is our go-to while we train. But if you cycle; run marathons, triathlons, or endurance races; or play a competitive recreational sport like tennis, you really need to dial in your hydration with carbohydrate and electrolytes. And if you're serious about it, I'd recommend a sports dietitian to help you individualize it.

Sports drinks can also be a good option if you train early in the morning and don't feel like eating much. A little carbohydrate and electrolytes can help you jump-start that workout and help you recover after a long training session. However, outside of physical exertion—hint: the name "sports drinks" should be a sign—these should not be your go-to drinks for daily hydration. They simply have too many unnecessary calories.

Energy drinks like Red Bull, Rockstar, and 5-hour Energy are predominantly caffeine, sweetener, and flavoring; some have ingredients like B vitamins thrown in. Specifically designed preworkout drinks may also have added amino acids to go along with their stimulant components, all designed to increase workout output. In preparation for and during activity, these drinks can prove effective. But they should be limited to those occasions and never used for regular consumption. Many pre-workout supplements, in fact, have the caffeine equivalent of several cups of coffee, along with added ingredients that can also speed up the central nervous system. It's like putting your energy level on steroids. All these stimulants can be dangerous for anyone but especially for those who are caffeine-sensitive. So it's critical not to abuse these drinks if you choose to use them as your source of energy before a workout.

BEER, WINE, AND ALCOHOL

A friend of mine at my gym came to me in a panic. He was working out hard and eating right but couldn't seem to shed any weight. He was beyond frustrated. We went over his daily routine and everything seemed to be on point for a healthy lifestyle. When I pressed him to think of anything he could be forgetting, he said: "Oh yeah, I drink up to a six-pack a few nights a week." That's like a guy in a sauna wondering why he can't stop sweating.

For some reason, many people don't appreciate how calorie-laden alcohol can be. My friend was sabotaging his efforts with a few thousand extra calories a week, yet it didn't even register as a problem. Beer is loaded with empty carbs. Not to mention, the more you drink, the less you care about what you eat. After a six-pack or bottle of wine, what's wrong with some ice cream with cookies or tacos at midnight? Plus, from a training standpoint, heavy alcohol consumption will impair muscle growth and affect recovery from workouts. Oh, and it dehydrates you. Yes, alcohol is the one fluid that does not count toward your daily fluid intake; in fact, it counts against it.

I'm not saying you need to refrain from all forms of adult beverages. I appreciate that drinking with friends or on social occasions can be fun, as well as offer a psychological release. Just make sure you're not doing it to mask unhappiness brought about by how you look and feel. Alcohol is a very short-term fix for that. In fact, eliminating alcohol as a crutch and getting in the best shape of your life is a surer path to solving those feelings of inadequacy.

But if you have a healthy relationship with alcohol and can responsibly enjoy it on a somewhat regular basis, you still need to do it in moderation. The American Heart Association suggests that alcohol consumption should be limited to one drink a day for women and two for men. Note that a drink is designated by appropriate serving sizes—for example, 5 ounces of red wine—not by the oversized novelty mug you got at the game. Certain drinks such as red wine have actually been shown to offer numerous benefits when consumed in this fashion. Tannins, which give red wine its color, have been linked to lowering coronary disease; resveratrol, a powerful antioxidant, protects against cell damage. Even beer in moderation has its pluses including anticancer properties, reduced risk of cardiovascular diseases and cognitive impairment, lowered blood pressure, and nutrients such as B-vitamins and folic acid.

All that said, if you don't drink now, I'm certainly not encouraging you to start. Even with some possible benefits, alcohol—especially hard liquor and spirits—doesn't constitute a health drink. There's still plenty of evidence that even moderate consumption has long-term drawbacks. And the 300 calories that a couple of beers can add to your daily total won't do much to flatten your stomach or pop your biceps. Drink enough of them, however, and it may still make you feel attractive.

So as you consider the numerous choices available, remember that all fluids, except alcohol, count toward your total daily fluid intake, but you don't want to be drinking many of your calories. If you enjoy a smoothie, include it; if you crave a glass of wine, don't deny yourself; if you juice, have at it. All can play a limited role in a smart nutrition plan. Just always pay attention that you are not going backward by downing an abundance of the calories you are working so hard to burn off.

DRINK RESPONSIBLY

Beverage	Approximate Calories	Running Distance Required to Burn It Off
Water	0 calories	0 miles
Large sweet tea	220 calories	2.25 miles
20-oz. bottle of soda	240 calories	2.5 miles
16-oz. Naked Juice Berry Blast	260 calories	2.75 miles
3 glasses of red wine	320 to 350 calories	3.5 miles
20-oz. Fruit Fusion smoothie	355 calories	3.5 miles
Venti mocha Frappuccino with whip	410 calories	4 miles
5 light beers	480 to 530 calories	5 miles
5 regular beers	750 calories	7.5 miles
Two 8-oz. frozen margaritas	800 to 1,200 calories	8 to 12 miles

CHAPTER 11
MEAL PLANNING

Nothing tastes as good as being fit feels.

Eating healthy on a consistent basis is not something most people can do overnight. To think that you are going to throw away every snack food in your refrigerator, never eat out again, and eat ten servings of vegetables every day when you have been doing none of that is pure fantasy. It's simply not going to happen. The key is to make small changes consistently until they become routine—choices like limiting desserts and alcohol to just weekends and special occasions, eliminating sugary soft drinks, and using mustard on sandwiches instead of mayonnaise. Then gradually add a few more small changes—such as replacing your processed cereal with homemade oatmeal, buying the leanest cuts of meat, and eating more fibrous vegetables at every meal—until the diet is significantly healthier and sustainable.

Yes, this requires discipline and sacrifice. But in the grand scheme of things you're getting off easy. In 2008 I went to Kenya on behalf of World Vision for a fact-finding mission to determine the needs of the people. There I saw young girls who should have been in grade school carrying buckets of water—sometimes on their heads!—for six hours every day because their village had none. I don't think it's asking too much to switch from ranch to spicy Dijon.

So start making changes. You may not be where you need to be yet, but you'll be closer than you were yesterday. It doesn't have to be perfect, and you will undoubtedly slip up on occasion—everybody does—but the key is to keep at it and continually make the best possible choices.

That's what this chapter is designed to show you. Just as you would in the gym, you need a detailed plan in the kitchen. If you walk into each day hoping the meals and snacks will just come together with no thought, magically cook themselves, and be ready to go in your work refrigerator to prevent you from going to a fast-food restaurant, you're also dreaming. If you're feeling that lucky, better get yourself some lottery tickets—you'll probably have just as good a chance of winning. Proper nutrition takes effort and foresight. And did I mention that third *D* in the 3D Body Revolution? *Discipline.* Lots and lots of discipline. Now that you've got the knowledge of what it takes to eat right, you've got to be vigilant to apply it. The eating plans laid out in this chapter will help by giving you daily meal suggestions with caloric guidelines based on the following simple principles:

- Eating small, frequent meals
- Consuming whole-grain carbohydrates or fruit with a lean protein at every meal and snack
- Garnishing meals and snacks with a healthy fat
- Eating as many nonstarchy vegetables as possible
- Hydrating with low-calorie beverages that don't fill your day with sugar and junk

This plan provides structure, but with choices. The meals and snacks have been arranged in this chapter, but you'll get to choose which ones you prefer based on availability and desire. Besides the examples here, dozens of additional recipes and snacks are presented in Chapter 12, broken down by meal and calorie count. The frequency of eating in this plan may be more than you're accustomed to. You may not be used to something like having a healthy snack an hour or so before going to sleep. You need to trust it.

It's really important to believe in the process, even if it doesn't make intuitive sense to you at first. When I first started performing on *Dancing with the Stars*, I was a bit reserved. I was a macho guy, and macho guys don't sway their hips. I was going to dance my own way and that would be good enough. My partner, Peta, and the coaches were constantly pushing me to stop judging myself and just let go. Smile, have fun, and allow myself to be vulnerable. Believe me, I thought I was way out of my league. But I bought into the process and improved every week on my way to winning the competition.

The goal is to start the day with a solid breakfast and then follow up with small frequent meals and snacks over the course of the day. Since you're never overly hungry, you will exhibit better portion control and be more likely to opt for healthier food choices at subsequent meals. This style of eating also encourages your energy levels to stay stable because your blood sugar resembles rolling hills instead of peaks and valleys—the ideal pattern. Skipping meals does not help you lose weight; it sets the stage for future feelings of starvation, which promote binge eating. And mind you, it will probably be a couple of slices of loaded pizza, not tilapia and broccoli.

But this is also not a restrictive diet; it's a healthy approach to nutrition that you can share and enjoy with your entire family. There's no need to have separate menus and shopping lists to satisfy your needs. That includes the occasional indulgence, because every food can fit into a lifestyle of healthy eating. It's called the 80/20 rule: 80 percent of the time, eat for your goal, be it to lose weight, have more energy, or get stronger in the weight room; 20 percent of the time you can eat for pleasure, including foods that are generally higher in fat, sugar, and calories, and lower in nutrients, but taste oh so good.

The following are sample daily meal plans based on three daily calorie ranges. Each is a template, but meals from the recipe section can be substituted so that a satisfying, individualized weekly plan can be formed. If you're looking to drop weight, you need to be in a caloric deficit; people looking to add muscle require a calorie surplus. Which brings us to the all-important question:

HOW MANY CALORIES SHOULD YOU BE EATING ON A DAILY BASIS?

The answer to this simple question depends on a variety of factors. Typically, a person's daily caloric requirement is calculated using height, weight, age, and, to get more exact, gender. That number, your resting metabolic rate, or RMR, is the number of calories you need to lie on the couch and simply occupy space. But since you're in no way going to resemble a couch potato, we have to include an Activity Factor—the amount of exercise you typically do over the course of a week—to see how many calories you need to maintain your weight (see chart, opposite). Then we can subtract calories to help you start losing weight, or add calories to the daily total if you want to gain muscle. From there, you can pick a meal plan and follow it.

Don't freak out; this simple formula will make it easy for you:

RMR = Weight in pounds × 10 = calories to be alive

RMR = _____ pounds × 10 = _____ calories

Calories to maintain weight = RMR calories × Activity Factor

_____ calories × _____ Activity Factor = _____ Total calories

Weight loss = Total calories − 500 = _____ calories to be eaten per day

Gain muscle = Total calories + 500 = _____ calories to be eaten per day

Women only = Total calories − 160 = _____ adjusted calories to be eaten per day

Example: 200-pound person working out 4 to 5 days a week wanting to lose weight

RMR = Weight in pounds × 10 = Calories to be alive

200 pounds × 10 = 2,000 calories

Calories to maintain weight = RMR calories × Activity Factor

2,000 calories × 1.4 Activity Factor = 2,750 total calories

Weight loss = Total calories − 500 = calories to be eaten per day

2,750 − 500 = 2,250 calories to be eaten per day

Women = 2,250 total calories − 160 = 2,090 calories to be eaten per day

ACTIVITY FACTOR CHART

Amount of Activity	Activity Factor
No exercise	1.2
1 to 3 days of exercise	1.3
3 to 5 days of exercise	1.4
5 to 6 days of exercise	1.5
6 days of exercise plus added workouts	1.7
Heavy training over 15 hours a week	1.9

Once you have calculated your calorie needs for your goal, then you can choose a meal plan that coincides appropriately. In the following meal plan examples, "c" indicates carbohydrate, "p" protein, and "f" fat. These calorie ranges are also a tool to use if you are making a recipe or dish that is not on the list, or when eating out. This is a template to make your new eating pattern easier and help it fit your life. Remember that the times and meals in the plan are a guide; you do not have to follow the times exactly, so rearrange the meals and snacks as you see fit. For example, you may eat a later breakfast if you work out in the morning, and then a later dinner; or your day might have breakfast, then lunch, with two snacks in the afternoon and a later dinner. So there's flexibility, but I don't want you skipping meals.

As the demands of the workout plans and calorie expenditure increase, so too can your daily caloric intake. Remember, if you want a car to run, you have to fuel it. And if you want your body to perform at the level you need it to while training on my programs, you have to fuel it with nutrient-rich meals and snacks over the course of the entire day. Skipping meals is like trying to drive a car that's running on empty—you'll be stumbling around, performing poorly, scrambling for whatever fuel you can find.

1,400- TO 1,600-CALORIE MEAL PLAN

Breakfast 6:00–8:00 a.m.	Snack 10:00–10:30 a.m.	Lunch 12:00–1:00 p.m.	Snack 3:30–4:30 p.m.	Dinner 6:00–8:00 p.m.	Snack 1–2 hours before bed
350 calories 30 c 20–25 p 8–10 f	150–200 calories 15–20 c 8–15 p 5–10 f	350 calories 30c 20–25 p 8–10 f	150–200 calories 15–20 c 8–15 p 5–10 f	350 calories 30 c 20–25 p 8–10 f	50–150 calories 10–20 c 5–10 p 0–5 f
½ cup (dry) oats Mix in 1 Tbsp. peanut/ almond butter 8 oz. low-fat milk **OR** 2–3 egg whites	½ mini whole wheat bagel **OR** 1 slice whole-wheat bread 1 Tbsp. peanut/ almond butter	Healthy quesadillas: 1 6" whole-wheat tortilla **OR** 2 corn tortillas ¼ cup 2% grated cheese 2–3 oz. chicken breast Fold over and broil in oven 1–2 mins./side ¼ cup guacamole/ avocado Salsa Salad with vegetables and dressing on side	Energy Bar: Luna, Clif MOJO, Larabar Alt, Zone, Pure Protein (small bar), Boundless Nutrition Oatmega Bar, Evolution Bar, Think Thin Bar, NuGo Thin Bar, KIND Bar + Protein	3 oz. meat—palm size (chicken, beef, pork, turkey, veggie patty) ½ cup carbohydrate (pasta, rice, potato, sweet potato, farro, couscous, quinoa, corn, peas, fruit) Salad with vegetables and dressing on side	6 oz. low-fat Greek yogurt ⅓ cup berries

If you are eating in this range, choose recipes from the 400-calorie-meal list. You can then add in two or three snacks over the course of the day.

1,600- TO 1,800-CALORIE MEAL PLAN

Breakfast 6:00–8:00 a.m.	Snack 10:00–10:30 a.m.	Lunch 12:00–1:00 p.m.	Snack 3:30–4:30 p.m.	Dinner 6:00–8:00 p.m.	Snack 1–2 hours before bed
400–450 calories 45 c 20–25 p 8–10 f	150–200 calories 25 c 10–15 p 5–10 f	400 calories 45 c 20–25 p 8–10 f	150–200 calories 25 c 10–15 p 5–10 f	450 calories 45 c 20–25 p 8–10 f	150 calories 15 c 10 p 5f
1 whole-wheat English muffin with 2 oz. lean Canadian bacon/ ham/turkey sausage, 1 slice 2% cheese, 1 egg 1 fruit	15 whole-wheat crackers with 2 oz. turkey	Sandwich on 2 slices whole-wheat/Ezekiel bread with 1 slice 2% cheese, 2 oz. meat, veggies, ¼ avocado 10 whole-wheat crackers **OR** pretzels Salad with vegetables and dressing on side	Homemade smoothie: 4 oz. vanilla yogurt, ½ scoop whey protein powder, ½ banana, 5 strawberries, ice and water to liking	3 oz. meat—palm size (chicken, fish, beef) 1–2 cups vegetables 1 cup carbohydrate (pasta, rice, potato, sweet potato, farro, couscous, quinoa, corn, peas, fruit) Salad with vegetables and dressing on side	1 slice Ezekiel bread with 1 Tbsp. peanut butter

If you are eating in this range, choose recipes from the 400-calorie-meal list. You can then add in three snacks over the course of the day. Or you can choose from the 500-calorie-meal list and have two snacks.

1,800- TO 2,000-CALORIE MEAL PLAN

Breakfast 6:00–8:00 a.m.	Snack 10:00–10:30 a.m.	Lunch 12:00–1:00 p.m.	Snack 3:30–4:30 p.m.	Dinner 6:00–8:00 p.m.	Snack 1–2 hours before bed
400–450 calories 45 c 25–33 p 10–15 f	200–250 calories 25 c 15 p 10 f	400 calories 45 c 20–25 p 8–10 f	200–250 calories 25 c 15 p 10 f	450–500 calories 45 c 25–30 p 8–12 f	150–200 calories 15–25 c 10 p 5 f
1 egg 2 slices turkey bacon 1 banana 6 oz. low-fat Greek yogurt with ½ cup berries and 1 Tbsp. chopped nuts	1 large apple with 1 Tbsp. peanut butter 1 hard-boiled egg	Sandwich on 2 slices Ezekiel bread with 3 oz. albacore tuna in water with veggies of choice, 1–2 Tbsp. avocado, 1 Tbsp. chopped pecans 1 fruit	½ cup low-fat cottage cheese ½ cup chopped fruit 2 Tbsp. chia seeds or flaxseeds	4 oz. meat—palm size (chicken, fish, turkey) 1–2 cups vegetables 1 cup carbohydrate (pasta, rice, potato, sweet potato, farro, couscous, quinoa, corn, peas, fruit) Salad with vegetables and dressing on side	6 oz. low-fat Greek yogurt ½ cup berries 5 almonds

If you are eating in this calorie range, choose recipes from the 500-calorie-meal list. You can then add in two or three snacks over the course of the day. Or you can choose from the 600-calorie-meal list and have one or two snacks.

If you calculate your calorie range needed for weight loss or muscle gain and find you need more calories—like our active 200-pound example who needs 2,250 calories a day—you can choose from the highest-calorie meal list and then add in snacks to help you reach your daily requirement. As mentioned, the meal plans have structure with choice so that you can individualize them and adapt them to your day.

EATING GUIDELINES FOR THE WORKOUT PLANS

BEGINNER

At this stage you're likely not burning an abundance of calories. So you need to be conservative with your calorie intake, especially if you want to lose weight and body fat. In order for those things to happen, you have to create a deficit of calories from what it takes to maintain your weight. The classic number is 500 calories less than you need, but you can adjust according to how you feel. Moving more and eating less equals pounds dropping. The meal plan is designed to provide small meals frequently to keep you from getting hungry. Remember, creating a deficit of calories means you may not feel full all the time, but that's okay. The goal is to hang out in hungry and satisfied, not starving and stuffed.

INTERMEDIATE

At this point, making healthy choices and exercising more regularly have become habits. Your workouts are getting more rigorous and likely occur more days a week. The increase in exercise typically means a greater nutritional demand for the body, but it also depends on your goal. If your intention is still weight loss and you have a decent amount to go, you can continue to limit your calorie intake. On the other hand, if you're more interested in maintaining weight and toning your muscles, consuming extra calories can add lean mass to your race-car frame.

ADVANCED

With elevated workout volume and intensity it is critically important to increase the number of calories you eat so that you have energy, can recover appropriately

Whether you like your current body weight or not, your body has nonetheless grown accustomed to it. That's where it feels most comfortable and ultimately wants to hang out. This is called the *set point theory*. Trying to deviate from that weight—up, or especially down—causes your body to react by maintaining your current weight, which is why weight loss is so difficult. So be aware that once you lose as little as 8 to 10 pounds, you may feel noticeably hungrier. That's your body trying to get back to its previously preferred weight. Don't fall into the trap. Hold tight a week and focus on drinking more water, filling up on nonstarchy, fiber-rich vegetables, and eating every few hours, and that feeling will eventually subside. You may have to use extra discipline and mind over matter— "I refuse to gain back the weight, I refuse to put on my fat pants"—but after a week to 10 days, your body will typically reset and create a new norm. Just stay focused on the goal and you will persevere. Remember: your body can stand almost anything. It's your mind that you have to convince. Eating healthy is a day-to-day decision. It may not always be the easiest decision, but long-term it's what helps you feel great and live a longer, healthier, and happier life.

after a workout, and are not starving over the course of the day. There's still room for variability based on goals such as weight loss and body composition, but at this training level you need the calories to support strenuous activity. However, this doesn't give you the green light to scarf down anything and everything. Choosing the highest-quality, least-processed options will help you noticeably lean out and detail your Porsche body with increased muscle definition.

CHAPTER 12

RECIPES

One of the very nicest things about life is the way we must regularly stop whatever it is we are doing and devote our attention to eating.

—Luciano Pavarotti

Eating well and treating your body right doesn't have to be complicated—these recipes prove that. They're broken down by calorie range and meal. While some take a little more effort and resources than others, none of them requires more than eight ingredients and 30 minutes—usually less—to put together. At the end (pages 194–211), there are some special recipes for the ambitious cook. Use any combination to create a savory meal plan that suits your caloric needs.

400- TO 500-CALORIE BREAKFASTS

THE BOWL

- ½ cup dry oats
- 1½ Tbsp. peanut butter **OR** 3 Tbsp. chopped nuts
- 6 oz. low-fat Greek yogurt

THE BREAKFAST SANDWICH

- 1 whole-wheat English muffin **OR** 2 slices double-fiber bread
- 2 to 3 oz. lean Canadian bacon/ham/ turkey sausage
- 1 slice 2% cheese
- 1 egg
- 1 fruit

THE BASIC BREAKFAST

- 1 egg and 2 egg whites, scrambled
- 2 slices turkey bacon
- 2 slices whole-wheat toast with thin-spread butter and cinnamon
- 6 oz. low-fat Greek yogurt

THE PARFAIT

- 6 oz. low-fat Greek yogurt
- 1 Tbsp. honey and 1 cup berries mixed in yogurt
- ¼ cup low-fat granola
- 2 eggs (on the side)

ON-THE-GO BREAKFAST

- 200-calorie energy bar
- 1 piece 2% string cheese
- 1 banana
- 10 to 15 almonds

400- TO 500-CALORIE LUNCHES

MIX-AND-MATCH

- 15 whole-wheat crackers
- 2 oz. lean deli meat
- 1 piece 2% string cheese
- 6 oz. low-fat Greek yogurt with ½ cup berries and ½ banana

PACK THE PITA

- 1 whole-wheat pita with 2 to 3 oz. chicken breast, ¼ cup 2% grated cheese, veggies, ⅓ avocado
- Side salad with dressing on side
- 1 fruit

OLD SCHOOL

- Peanut butter (2 Tbsp.) and jelly (1 Tbsp.) sandwich on whole-wheat bread
- 1 fruit

GO FISH

- 3 oz. albacore tuna in water with 1 Tbsp. light mayo and some mustard, veggies of choice, and 1 Tbsp. chopped pecans
- 2 slices whole-wheat bread or 15 whole-wheat crackers
- 1 small fruit **OR** ½ cup chopped fruit

WRAP IT UP

- The wrap:
  - 1 whole-wheat tortilla
  - 3 oz. grilled chicken breast
  - Veggies
  - 1 slice 2% cheese **OR** ¼ cup grated 2% cheese
  - 1 to 2 Tbsp. hummus
  - 10 whole-wheat crackers
  - Salad with dressing on side

400- TO 500-CALORIE DINNERS

THE BASIC

- 4 oz. meat—palm size (chicken, fish, beef, pork, turkey)
- 1 to 2 cups vegetables
- 1 cup carbohydrate (pasta, rice, potato, sweet potato, quinoa, couscous, corn, fruit, bread)
- Side salad with dressing on side

STIR-FRY

- *Mix together the following:*
  - 4 oz. grilled chicken breast
  - 2 to 3 cups sautéed vegetables
  - 1 cup brown rice
  - Soy sauce to taste

TACO SALAD

- 3 to 5 cups lettuce and veggies
- ¼ cup 2% grated cheese
- 1 cup ground turkey meat browned on the stove with taco seasoning
- ¼ cup yellow corn **OR** black beans
- ½ cup guacamole
- 8 light tortilla chips crumbled in
- Salsa

PITA PIZZA

- *Top the pita with tomato sauce, cheese, and meat. Broil in oven for 4 to 5 minutes.*
  - 1 whole-wheat pita
  - ¼ cup tomato sauce
  - ⅓ cup 2% grated cheese
  - 2 to 3 oz. chicken **OR** turkey **OR** turkey sausage
- Salad with 2 Tbsp. dried fruit, 2 Tbsp. nuts, and dressing on side

BURGER BASH

- 100% whole-wheat hamburger bun
- 4 oz. lean ground meat patty
- Veggies
- 1 to 2 Tbsp. smashed avocado
- Big salad with lots of veggies, 2 Tbsp. nuts, and dressing on side

500- TO 600-CALORIE BREAKFASTS

WAFFLE IRON

- 2 whole-wheat waffles
- 1 Tbsp. peanut butter spread on each waffle (can add cinnamon)
- 8 oz. low-fat milk with ½ scoop whey protein powder

ANY-DAY EGG SANDWICH

- 1 whole-wheat English muffin
- 3 oz. lean Canadian bacon
- 1 slice 2% cheese
- 1 egg
- 4 oz. low-fat Greek yogurt with ¼ cup low-fat granola

THIS-AND-THAT

- 1 egg and 2 egg whites, scrambled with veggies
- 1 slice whole-wheat toast with 1 Tbsp. peanut butter
- ½ cup berries
- 8 oz. low-fat milk with ½ scoop protein powder

SMOOTHIE

- 1 scoop whey protein
- 4 oz. low-fat vanilla Greek yogurt
- 8 oz. low-fat milk
- 1 banana
- ½ cup berries
- 1 Tbsp. almond butter

CEREAL COMBO

- 2 eggs with veggies
- 1¼ cups whole-grain cereal with low-fat milk
- 1 banana
- 8 oz. low-fat milk

500- TO 600-CALORIE LUNCHES

HIGH-PROTEIN WRAP

- The wrap:
    - ⅓ cup grated 2% cheese
    - 3 to 4 oz. lean meat
    - Veggies
    - 1 Tbsp. hummus or vinaigrette
- 1 cup strawberries and 8 to 10 grapes
- 15 whole-wheat crackers **OR** pretzels

TACO TUESDAY

- The tacos:
    - 2 6-inch white corn tortillas
    - 2 oz. grilled mahi-mahi
    - 1 to 2 Tbsp. Mexican cheese
    - ¼ cup black beans
    - ¼ avocado
- Salad with ¼ cup corn, tomato, red bell pepper, and dressing on side

WARM SALMON SALAD

- 2 cups sautéed spinach, sautéed lightly with olive oil
- ½ bag Tasty Bite Multigrain Pilaf
- 4 to 5 oz. grilled salmon

BROWN BAG

- The sandwich:
    - 2 slices whole-wheat bread
    - 1 slice 2% cheese
    - 4 oz. lean meat
    - Veggies
    - 2 Tbsp. hummus
- 10 whole-wheat crackers **OR** pretzels
- 1 cup chopped fruit **OR** banana

THE SNACK BAGGIE

- ½ peanut butter and jelly sandwich with 1 Tbsp. peanut butter and 1 Tbsp. jelly
- 10 whole-wheat crackers **OR** pretzels
- 6 oz. low-fat Greek yogurt with ¼ cup granola and ½ cup chopped fruit
- 1 piece 2% string cheese

500- TO 600-CALORIE DINNERS

THE BASIC

- 5 oz. meat—palm size (chicken, fish, beef, pork, turkey)
- 1 to 2 cups vegetables
- 1 cup carbohydrate (pasta, rice, potato, sweet potato, quinoa, couscous, corn, fruit, bread)
- Side salad with dressing on side

GO GREEN

- Big salad with mixed greens and veggies
- 5 oz. grilled chicken breast
- 3 Tbsp. nuts, ½ cup chopped berries
- Dressing on side
- 1 large sweet potato baked with skin on and drizzled with olive oil

CHICKEN PARMESAN

- 5 oz. chicken breast breaded with egg white, Italian-seasoned bread crumbs, and 2 Tbsp. reduced-fat Parmesan cheese
- 1¼ cups spinach pasta, cooked al dente and topped with ½ cup Healthy Choice tomato sauce
- 1 cup fresh spinach mixed with cooked pasta
- 2 cups Italian vegetables (veggies of choice baked in oven with Italian seasoning)

THE SHROOM

- Stuff 2 grilled portabella mushrooms with:
  - 2½ oz. chicken
  - Veggies of choice (cooked lightly in extra-virgin olive oil)
  - ¾ cup brown rice **OR** whole-grain rice pilaf
- Salad with veggies and dressing on side

HEALTHY QUESADILLA

- The quesadilla:
  - 1 whole-wheat tortilla
  - ½ cup 2% grated cheese
  - 5 oz. chopped cooked chicken breast (*Fold over and broil in oven for 2 minutes per side.*)
  - ⅓ avocado
- 10 light tortilla chips and salsa
- Side salad with dressing on side

CLEAN BREAKFAST

- 2 cups fruit
- 1 egg
- 1 cup low-fat cottage cheese
- 15 to 20 almonds

THE REAL BACON DEAL

- 2 eggs with a sprinkle of 2% grated cheese
- 3 to 4 slices bacon
- 2 slices whole-wheat toast with 1 Tbsp. 100% fruit jelly on each slice
- 1 fruit
- 8 oz. low-fat milk

OATS AND MORE

- The oats:
  - 1 cup steel-cut oats
  - 1 Tbsp. honey
  - ¼ cup fruit
  - 1½ Tbsp. natural peanut butter
- 1 egg and 3 egg whites, scrambled

SMOOTHIE SATISFACTION

- 1 scoop whey protein
- 8 oz. low-fat milk
- 4 oz. low-fat Greek yogurt
- 1 cup berries
- 2 Tbsp. honey
- 2 Tbsp. uncooked oats
- 1 Tbsp. peanut butter

QUICK BITES

- Peanut butter balls (*Mix together, roll into 24 balls, and refrigerate.*):
  - ½ cup peanut butter
  - ¼ cup honey
  - 1 cup oats
  - ½ cup whey protein powder
- 1 banana
- 16 oz. low-fat milk

ROLL-UPS

- The roll-ups:
  - two 6-inch whole-wheat tortillas
  - 5 to 6 oz. lean deli meat
  - 2 oz. 2% cheese
  - All sorts of veggies
- 1 fruit

THE BASIC BIGGER LUNCH

- The sandwich:
  - 2 slices whole-wheat bread
  - 1 slice 2% Swiss cheese
  - 6 oz. smoked turkey
  - Veggies
  - Pesto, for drizzling
- 15 whole-wheat crackers **OR** pretzels
- 1 fruit
- 10 almonds

GRILLED CHEESE

- The sandwich:
  - 2 slices whole-wheat bread, toasted in a pan with 1 to 2 Tbsp. yogurt-based butter

- 2 slices 2% cheese
- 3 oz. lean ham
- 150-to-200-calorie serving tomato soup

TWISTED PHILLY CHEESE BAGEL

- The bagel:
  - 1 whole-wheat bagel
  - 4 oz. lean roast beef
  - 1 slice 2% provolone cheese
- 1 apple, sliced, covered in cinnamon, and microwaved until soft, then drizzled with 4 oz. low-fat vanilla Greek yogurt

TUNA MELT

- The melt:
  - 2 whole-wheat English muffins, toasted
  - 2 oz. tuna (water-packed)
  - 1 slice 2% Swiss cheese (melted)
  - Veggies of choice
- ½ to 1 cup chopped fruit

SIMPLE DINNER

- 7 oz. meat—palm size (chicken, fish, beef, pork, turkey)
- 2 cups vegetables drizzled with extra-virgin olive oil
- ½ cup carbohydrate (rice, pasta, potato, quinoa, fruit, beans, corn, bread)
- Side salad with dressing on side

GO LEAN

- Big salad with 7 oz. grilled chicken breast, 3 Tbsp. nuts, and ½ cup mandarin oranges
- 1 large fruit **OR** 1¼ cup chopped fruit
- 2 slices whole-wheat bread/toast **OR** 15 whole-wheat crackers

LETTUCE WRAPS

- Wrap filling:
  - 7 oz. diced chicken cooked with water chestnuts, chives, and vegetables of choice
  - Soy sauce to taste
- Large iceberg lettuce leaves (for wrapping)
- 1½ cups brown rice

BREAKFAST FOR DINNER

- The wrap:
  - 2 whole-wheat tortillas
  - 1 egg and 3 egg whites, scrambled
  - ¼ cup 2% cheese and veggies
- 1 fruit

SALMON SLIDERS

- The sliders:
  - 3 mini slider buns (whole-wheat, if possible)
  - 2 oz. salmon
  - Spinach and a slice of tomato
  - Grilled onions
  - 1 tsp. pesto mayo
- Mixed green salad with dressing on side

CHEAT MEALS

As explained earlier, I want you to subscribe to the 80/20 rule. That means that four out of five meals are safely in your calorie range, with the right kinds of foods present. Basically it's the meals and snacks found in the recipes. That fifth meal? That's where you can have a little fun. These "cheat meals" give you latitude to enjoy foods that generally don't fall in the healthy category. But savory food is one of life's pleasures, and any realistic eating plan designed for long-term success needs to make allowances for it. And nobody likes the guy who brings his own salad to a Super Bowl party. There's even some theory that the occasional cheat meal during a consistent caloric deficit prevents the body from going into starvation mode, encouraging it to continually burn fat stores.

You'll notice, however, that I have not provided recipes for cheat meals. My experience is that most people don't need my help in this department. You can certainly super-size any of the recipes by adding a side of fries or chips to burgers and sandwiches, hash browns and bacon to an omelet, or an extra quesadilla on taco night. But I leave the details in your capable hands. If you have any doubts whether something is a cheat meal, then it probably is. I equate it to that old definition of pornography: you know it when you see it.

That said, I want to offer a couple of cheat meal guidelines. First, if you don't want to indulge, then don't. If you're enjoying the meal plan and have been experiencing noticeable improvement in your energy level and pounds are dripping off your body, there's no reason to slow it down. Stay on that righteous path. Space your cheats out even further for the rare piece of birthday cake, slice of pecan pie at Thanksgiving, or drinks and apps at a wedding reception cocktail hour.

Second, if you're going to cheat on your meal plan, don't be a serial adulterer. The bigger and more frequent your strays from clean eating—it's a cheat meal, not a cheat day—the more difficult it will be to reach your goals. You may derail your efforts entirely. Remember, this is an opportunity to eat some of the foods you like, not a license to clean out your refrigerator or order everything on the right side of the menu. It doesn't hurt to buffer the extra calories by cutting back on other meals—a smaller breakfast or lunch, skipping a snack—when you know a cheat is on the way. But you also don't want to be famished heading into a cheat meal, because then you can really go to hell with yourself. Also, try to keep the cheats as nutrient-filled as possible. An extra sushi roll or a thick piece of roasted veggie lasagna are lesser evils than a box of Krispy Kreme doughnuts or a pint of Ben & Jerry's. Use the cheat as a way to satisfy a craving, not put your head in a trough.

150- TO 250-CALORIE SNACKS

Each contains 15 to 25 grams carbohydrate, 8 to 12 grams protein, and 5 to 10 grams fat.

Energy Bar: Luna, Luna Protein, Zone, Clif MOJO, Larabar, Pure Protein (small bar), Boundless Nutrition Omega-3 Bar, Evolution Bar (Starbucks/Whole Foods), Think Thin Bar, NuGo Thin Bar, Power Crunch bar	½ mini whole-wheat bagel **OR** 1 slice whole-wheat/ Ezekiel bread with 1 Tbsp. peanut/ almond butter 4 oz. low-fat milk	3 peanut/almond butter balls: ½ cup peanut/ almond butter ¼ cup honey 1 cup oats ½ cup whey protein powder Mix peanut butter and honey; then stir in oats and whey powder. Roll into 24 balls and refrigerate.	12 oz. low-fat milk 10 almonds
1 apple with 1 Tbsp. peanut/almond butter 4 oz. low-fat Greek yogurt	100-calorie microwave popcorn 1 oz. 2% cheese	Homemade trail mix: ½ cup whole-grain cereal, 1 Tbsp. dried fruit, 10 nuts 4 oz. low-fat Greek yogurt	1 apple, chopped and covered in cinnamon; warm in the microwave for 2 minutes Top with light vanilla Greek yogurt and 2 Tbsp. flaxseeds

6 oz. low-fat Greek yogurt with ½ cup berries and 2 Tbsp. nuts	Kashi TLC Chewy granola bar **OR** Fiber One granola bar 4 oz. low-fat Greek yogurt **OR** cottage cheese	1 whole-wheat tortilla 1½ oz. 2% cheese	20 grapes 1.5 oz. 2% cheese
½ whole-wheat English muffin with 1½ oz. 2% cheese	10 whole-wheat crackers 1 piece 2% string cheese 2 Tbsp. hummus	2 oz. lean meat 1 fruit 12 almonds	1 pack peanut butter crackers 4 oz. low-fat Greek yogurt **OR** beef jerky stick
12 almonds 1 fruit 6 oz. low-fat Greek yogurt	1 hard-boiled egg 1 piece 2% string cheese 1 fruit	10 to 12 oz. skinny latte 1 fruit	12 whole-wheat crackers ¼ avocado 2 oz. turkey/ chicken

CHILI-RUBBED TILAPIA WITH ASPARAGUS AND LEMON

1. Bring 1 inch of water to a boil in a large saucepan. Put the asparagus in a steamer basket, place in the pan, cover, and steam until crisp-tender, about 4 minutes. Transfer to a large plate, spreading out to cool.

2. Combine the chili powder, garlic powder, and ¼ tsp. of the salt on a plate. Dredge the fillets in the spice mixture to coat.

3. Heat the oil in a large nonstick skillet over medium-high heat. Add the fish and cook until just opaque in the center, gently turning halfway, 5 to 7 minutes total. Divide among 4 plates.

4. Immediately add the lemon juice, the remaining ¼ tsp. salt, and the asparagus to the pan and cook, stirring constantly, until the asparagus is coated and heated through, about 2 minutes. Serve the asparagus with the fish.

Serves 4

2 lbs. asparagus, tough ends trimmed, cut into 1-inch pieces

2 Tbsp. chili powder

½ tsp. garlic powder

½ tsp. salt

1 lb. tilapia, Pacific sole, or other firm whitefish fillets

2 Tbsp. extra-virgin olive oil

¼ cup lemon juice

CHICKEN CAESAR PASTA SALAD

1. Bring a large pot of water to a boil. Cook the pasta according to the package directions. Drain and set aside.

2. Preheat a grill pan over high heat. Pat the chicken dry and cut into strips. Season with salt, pepper, and paprika. Grill on both sides until done, about 5 minutes. Let cool and then slice into bite-size pieces.

3. To make the dressing, whisk all the ingredients together in a small bowl until you achieve a creamy consistency.

4. If you are making your own croutons, cut the slice of bread into small cubes and dry-fry in a nonstick frying pan over medium heat until golden and crispy, about 5 minutes.

5. To assemble the salad, put the pasta and chicken into a large bowl. Add the lettuce and tomatoes. Pour in the dressing and toss until evenly coated. Top with the croutons and serve immediately.

Serves 4

7 oz. whole-wheat pasta, preferably small shapes

12 oz. boneless, skinless chicken breasts

Salt and freshly ground black pepper

Paprika

4 heads romaine lettuce, shredded

1 pint cherry tomatoes, halved

DRESSING

4 Tbsp. low-fat Greek yogurt

4 Tbsp. lemon juice

2 Tbsp. grated Parmesan

2 tsp. Dijon mustard

Salt and freshly ground black pepper

CROUTONS

1 slice whole-grain bread or 4 Tbsp. store-bought croutons

SOLE AND SUMMER VEGETABLE PARCHMENT PACKETS

1. Preheat the oven to 325°F. In a small bowl, stir together the butter, shallot, 2 Tbsp. of the chives, and the lemon zest, salt, and pepper. In a saucepan, prepare the rice according to package directions, adding 1 Tbsp. of the butter mixture to the saucepan along with the rice.

2. Meanwhile, coat the fish with the remaining butter mixture. Arrange four 5-inch-long sheets of parchment paper on a work surface with the long end closest to you. Pile 1 cup of the spinach in the center of one sheet. Arrange 2 fish pieces, side by side, vertically in the center of the spinach. Lay ¼ each of the zucchini, carrot, and bell pepper crosswise over the fish. Roll both fish pieces upward over the vegetables to form a bundle. Arrange the bundle seam side down in the center of the parchment. Fold in the long sides and then the short sides of the parchment, pressing the edges as you fold to form a package.

3. Repeat with the remaining ingredients to create four packets. Arrange on a rimmed baking sheet. Bake until the fish flakes easily when tested with a

Serves 4

¼ cup organic unsalted butter, softened

1 small shallot, minced

3 Tbsp. chopped fresh chives

Zest and juice of 1 lemon

¾ tsp. sea salt

¼ tsp. freshly ground black pepper

⅔ cup long-grain brown rice, rinsed

1 lb. boneless, skinless sole fillets, cut into 8 pieces and patted dry

4 cups baby spinach

1 zucchini, cut into 2-inch matchsticks

1 carrot, cut into 2-inch matchsticks

1 red or yellow bell pepper, cut into 2-inch matchsticks

fork, the spinach is bright green, and the vegetables are crisp-tender, about 15 minutes.

4. Divide the rice among 4 plates. Carefully open the parchment packets. Using a slotted spoon, divide the spinach and fish among the plates, pouring any juices from the packets over the top. Drizzle with lemon juice and sprinkle with the remaining 1 Tbsp. chives.

BAKED CHICKEN BREASTS WITH DIJON–WHITE WINE SAUCE AND HARICOTS VERTS

1. Preheat the oven to 425°F.

2. Heat a large ovenproof skillet over medium-high heat. Add the oil and swirl to coat the pan. Sprinkle the chicken with salt and pepper. Add the chicken to the pan and cook browned, about 5 minutes. Turn the chicken over and place the pan in the oven. Bake until cooked through, 7 to 8 minutes. Remove the pan from the oven. Place the chicken on a plate and cover to keep warm.

3. Return the pan to the stove over medium heat. Add the carrots, shallots, thyme, and garlic and sauté for 2 minutes. Add the wine to pan; cook for 2 minutes or until the liquid is reduced by half, scraping the pan to loosen the browned bits. Add the stock to pan and cook until slightly thickened, about 2 minutes. Stir in the clarified butter and mustard.

4. Bring a large saucepan of water to a boil. Add the haricots verts and cook until crisp-tender, about 4 minutes. Drain. Toss the haricots verts with a sprinkle of salt and pepper and serve with the chicken and sauce.

Serves 4

3 tsp. grapeseed oil

4 to 6 oz. boneless, skinless chicken breast halves

½ tsp. sea salt

½ tsp. freshly ground black pepper

½ cup diced carrots

4 Tbsp. thinly sliced shallots

2 tsp. chopped fresh thyme

3 garlic cloves, chopped

½ to ¾ cup white wine

¾ cup chicken stock

2 Tbsp. clarified butter (ghee)

2 tsp. Dijon mustard

1 pound haricots verts (green beans), trimmed

HERBED TURKEY SCALLOPINE
WITH LEMON-DIJON KALE

1. In a small bowl, combine the flour, dill, sesame seeds, paprika, salt, and pepper; sprinkle all over turkey, patting to coat.

2. Coat a large heavy skillet with cooking spray and heat over medium. In two batches, add the turkey and cook, turning once, until lightly golden and just cooked through, 3 to 4 minutes per batch. Transfer to a plate. Wipe out the skillet and coat with cooking spray; return to medium heat. Add the onion and garlic and sauté, stirring frequently, until softened, about 2 minutes.

3. Add the broth, mustard, and lemon zest and stir until combined; stir in the kale. Bring to a boil over medium-high heat; then reduce the heat to medium-low, cover, and simmer until the kale is tender and the sauce has thickened slightly, 3 to 4 minutes.

4. Return the turkey to skillet in a single layer over the top of the kale. Cover and simmer until the turkey is heated through, 1 to 2 minutes. Divide the turkey and kale among 6 plates and sprinkle with hazelnuts, if desired.

Serves 6

3 Tbsp. whole-wheat flour

2 Tbsp. chopped fresh dill

2 tsp. sesame seeds

½ tsp. paprika

¼ tsp. sea salt

¼ tsp. freshly ground black pepper

1 lb. turkey breast scallopine, cut into 6 pieces

Olive oil cooking spray

½ red onion, thinly sliced

2 garlic cloves, thinly sliced

2½ cups low-sodium chicken broth

1½ Tbsp. grainy or Dijon mustard

1½ tsp. lemon zest

8 cups sliced kale leaves (in ribbons), tough stems removed

⅓ cup sliced or chopped toasted hazelnuts (optional)

GLAZED SALMON AND RICE BOWL WITH SNOW PEAS

1. Whisk the soy sauce, 1 Tbsp. of the vinegar, and the honey in a small bowl. Place half of the honey mixture and the salmon in a large zip-top bag, seal, and refrigerate for 15 to 20 minutes. Reserve the remaining honey mixture.

2. Remove the salmon from the marinade; discard the marinade. Heat a grill pan or sauté pan over medium heat. Coat the pan with cooking spray and add the salmon, skin side up; cook to the desired degree of doneness, about 3 minutes on each side. Remove the salmon from the pan.

3. Prepare the rice and peas according to package instructions. Divide the rice and peas among 4 bowls; top evenly with the salmon. Drizzle the reserved honey mixture over the salmon and sprinkle with sesame seeds and scallions.

Serves 4

3 Tbsp. low-sodium soy sauce

3 Tbsp. rice vinegar

2 Tbsp. raw honey

4 6-oz. skin-on salmon fillets

Cooking spray

1 8½-ounce pouch precooked brown rice

1 8- to 10-ounce bag snow peas or sugar snap peas (steam-in-the-bag)

1 Tbsp. toasted sesame seeds

½ cup chopped scallions, white and green parts

ROASTED PORK TENDERLOIN WITH BUTTERNUT SQUASH, KALE, AND TOMATOES

1. Preheat the oven to 300°F.

2. Combine the paprika, garam masala, garlic powder, onion powder, salt, and pepper in a small bowl. Add the lemon juice and stir. Place the pork in a Dutch oven or deep roasting pan and coat all sides of the pork with the spice mixture.

3. Add 1 cup of the stock and cover tightly with a lid or foil. Roast in the oven for at least 2 hours, turning the pork over every 45 minutes.

4. After at least 2 hours, add the squash and the remaining ½ cup stock. Return the pan to the oven and roast for 30 minutes more; then add the kale and tomatoes. Return the pan to the oven and roast for 15 minutes more.

5. Remove the pan from the oven and leave uncovered until ready to serve. Arrange the vegetables on 4 plates and break the pork apart into chunks and place over the vegetables. Spoon the liquid from the pan over the pork.

Serves 4

2 tsp. smoked paprika

2 tsp. garam masala

1 tsp. garlic powder

1 tsp. onion powder

1 tsp. sea salt or kosher salt

½ tsp. freshly ground black pepper

Juice of ½ lemon

1½ to 2 lbs. boneless pork tenderloin

1½ cups chicken stock or water

1 butternut squash, diced into 1-inch cubes

Bunch of kale, stems removed and leaves chopped

1 cup fire-roasted diced tomatoes

FLANK STEAK WITH HERB DRESSING AND CHARRED BROCCOLINI

1. Combine 3 Tbsp. of the oil, 3 Tbsp. of the herbs, and the garlic in a skillet over medium heat. Cook for 2 minutes, stirring frequently. Remove the mixture from the pan and place in a bowl.

2. Cut the steak into 4 equal pieces and sprinkle each piece with salt and pepper. Return the pan to medium heat and add the steak to the pan. Cook to the desired degree of doneness, about 4 minutes on each side. Remove the steak from the pan and place it in a shallow dish to collect the juices; then sprinkle it with the remaining 1 Tbsp. herbs.

3. Return the pan to medium heat and add the remaining 1 Tbsp. oil to the pan. Add the broccolini and cook for 2 minutes. Add ½ cup water to the pan, cover, and cook until tender, about 3 minutes. Sprinkle with salt and drizzle with lemon juice.

4. Divide the steak among 4 plates. Whisk the steak juices and herb mixture together. Serve the steak with the herb dressing and broccolini.

Serves 4

¼ cup extra-virgin olive oil

¼ cup finely chopped fresh poultry herb blend

2 tsp. minced fresh garlic

1 lb. flank steak

¾ tsp. sea salt

½ tsp. freshly ground black pepper

1 lb. broccolini, trimmed and cut into 1-inch pieces

2 tsp. lemon juice

BBQ CHICKEN WITH ROASTED BRUSSELS SPROUTS AND CARROTS

1. In a large bowl, whisk together the ketchup, chile, honey, cumin, and garlic. Add the chicken and toss to coat. Cover and refrigerate for 2 hours or overnight.

2. Preheat the oven to 425°F. Line a large rimmed baking sheet with foil or parchment paper. Arrange the chicken in a single layer on half of the sheet. In a separate large bowl, toss together the Brussels sprouts, shallot, carrot, and oil.

3. Spread the vegetables in a single layer on the remaining half of the sheet. Sprinkle the chicken and vegetables with salt and pepper.

4. Bake until the juices run clear when the chicken is pierced, an instant-read thermometer reads 165°F when inserted in the thickest part of the meat, and the vegetables are tender and browned, about 30 minutes.

5. Divide the chicken and vegetables among 4 plates and serve.

Serves 4

½ cup ketchup

1½ Tbsp. chopped chipotle chile in adobo sauce

1½ Tbsp. raw honey

1 tsp. ground cumin

1 garlic clove, crushed

8 chicken drumsticks (2 lbs.), skin removed

1½ lbs. Brussels sprouts, trimmed and halved

1 large shallot, cut into 1-inch-thick wedges

1 carrot, sliced diagonally into ¼-inch rounds

2 Tbsp. extra-virgin olive oil

½ tsp. salt

½ tsp. freshly ground black pepper

PEACH-GLAZED TURKEY BREAST (TENDERLOIN) WITH MUSTARD GREENS

1. Season the turkey with salt and pepper. In a heavy 12-inch skillet, heat the oil over medium heat. Add the turkey, skin side up, and cook undisturbed until golden brown, 6 to 7 minutes. Turn the turkey over and arrange along the outer edge of the skillet. Add the parsnip to the center of the skillet in a single layer. Cook undisturbed until it begins to brown, 2 to 3 minutes.

2. In a small bowl, whisk together the stock, maple syrup, vinegar, and mustard and stir into the skillet. Stir in the peach and reduce the heat to low. Cover and cook undisturbed until the peach is softened and an instant-read thermometer reads 165°F when inserted in the thickest part of the meat, 15 to 17 minutes.

3. Meanwhile, bring a saucepan of water to a boil. Add the mustard greens and cook until bright green, about 30 seconds. Drain well and pat dry or whirl the greens in a salad spinner.

4. Stir the greens into the turkey mixture. Increase the heat to medium and cook, uncovered, basting the turkey with sauce occasionally, until the sauce is thickened, 3 to 5 minutes. Divide between 2 plates and serve.

Serves 2

2 turkey breasts (tenderloin), trimmed

Salt and freshly ground black pepper

2 tsp. extra-virgin olive oil

1 large parsnip, peeled, quartered lengthwise, and sliced crosswise into 1-inch lengths

¼ cup chicken stock

2 Tbsp. pure maple syrup

1 Tbsp. apple cider vinegar

2 tsp. Dijon mustard

1 large peach, peeled, pitted, and chopped, or 2 cups frozen diced peaches, thawed and drained

10 oz. mustard greens, thick stems removed and leaves torn (about 12 cups)

LEMON CHICKEN WITH SAUTÉED SQUASH AND SWEET POTATO MEDLEY

1. Preheat the oven to 350°F. In a medium bowl, combine ⅓ cup of the rosemary with the fennel seeds, 1½ tsp. of the pepper, the garlic, lemon juice, soy sauce, and 2 Tbsp. of the oil.

2. Place the chicken in a roasting pan, breast side up. Gently slide your fingers under the skin and rub in a thick layer of the rosemary mixture, leaving the skin on. Spread the remaining rosemary mixture in the chicken cavity and place the lemon rind inside.

3. Roast the chicken for 2½ hours or until an instant-read thermometer reads 165°F when inserted in the inner thigh. Remove from the oven, tent with foil, and let rest for 10 minutes.

4. Near the end of the roasting time, prepare the sweet potato medley. Heat the remaining 4 tsp. oil in a large skillet over medium-high heat. Add the potatoes and the remaining 2 Tbsp. rosemary and sauté for 5 minutes; cover and cook for 8 minutes more. Stir in the onion, zucchini, yellow squash, and the remaining ½ tsp. pepper. Cover and cook until the squash is softened, 7 to 8 minutes.

5. When done, remove the sweet potato–squash medley and evenly divide among 6 plates. Remove the skin from chicken, slice the meat, and add to the top of vegetable medley.

Serves 6

⅓ cup plus 2 Tbsp. chopped fresh rosemary leaves

3 Tbsp. dried fennel seeds

2 tsp. freshly ground black pepper

5 garlic cloves, minced

¼ cup fresh lemon juice (reserve rind)

2 Tbsp. low-sodium soy sauce

2 Tbsp. plus 4 tsp. extra-virgin olive oil

1 8-lb. whole chicken (giblets removed), rinsed and patted dry

3 small sweet potatoes, scrubbed and chopped into ¼-inch pieces

1 yellow onion, chopped into ¼-inch pieces

2 small zucchini, chopped into ¼-inch pieces

2 small yellow squash, chopped into ¼-inch pieces

CHICKEN, SAUSAGE, AND SHRIMP GUMBO AND BROWN RICE

1. Cook the brown rice according to package directions.

2. In a large soup pot over medium heat, heat 2 Tbsp. of the oil. Add the sausage and brown on all sides, cooking through. Remove to a plate to rest and slice it into bite-size pieces.

3. Add the remaining ½ cup oil and the flour to the pot, stirring to combine. Cook over medium to medium-low heat, stirring often and scraping the bottom of the pan, until the mixture (roux) turns the color of dark peanut butter or even a little darker, about 8 minutes.

4. Increase the heat to medium-high. Add the onion, celery, and bell pepper to the roux, stirring to combine. Add salt and pepper and the cayenne. Cook until the vegetables soften, 5 to 10 minutes.

5. Add the beer and stir, scraping the bits off the bottom of the pot. Add the stock, stirring to combine. Reduce the heat to low.

6. Add the reserved sausage and the chicken and bay leaves. Simmer until the chicken is cooked through, about 1 hour. Add the shrimp and cook until the shrimp are cooked, 5 to 10 minutes.

7. Serve the gumbo over the rice.

Serves 6

2 cups uncooked brown rice

½ cup plus 2 Tbsp. grapeseed oil

4 links turkey sausage

½ cup all-purpose flour

1 cup diced onion

½ cup diced celery

½ cup diced green bell pepper

Sea salt and freshly ground black pepper

1 tsp. cayenne pepper

1 cup beer

3 cups chicken stock

2 lbs. boneless, skinless chicken breasts

3 bay leaves

1 lb. shrimp, peeled and deveined

CREAMY CHICKEN BIRYANI

1. In a large deep skillet or Dutch oven with a tight-fitting lid, heat the oil over medium heat. Add the onion and cook, stirring frequently, until softened, about 5 minutes. Add the garam masala, turmeric, and red pepper flakes and cook, stirring gently, 30 to 45 seconds. Add the garlic, tomatoes, and ginger. Cook, stirring frequently, until the tomato has broken down slightly, about 5 minutes.

2. Add the yogurt, stirring to combine into a thick paste. Add the chicken, reduce the heat to medium-low, cover, and simmer until the sauce is slightly reduced, about 10 minutes.

3. Add the cauliflower, replace the lid, and continue cooking until the cauliflower is tender and the chicken is no longer pink inside, 10 to 15 minutes. Divide among 4 plates and garnish with fresh mint.

Serves 4

1 Tbsp. grapeseed oil

1 red onion, diced

1 Tbsp. garam masala

½ to 1 tsp. ground turmeric

½ to 1 tsp. crushed red pepper flakes

3 garlic cloves, roasted and minced

2 cups roasted diced tomatoes with juices

1 Tbsp. grated fresh ginger

1 cup whole-milk yogurt (nonfat yogurt most likely would curdle in this dish)

1 lb. boneless chicken breast (skin on or off as desired), chopped into 1-inch chunks

2 cups cauliflower florets

1 Tbsp. chopped fresh mint leaves

CREAMY CHICKEN QUINOA AND BROCCOLI CASSEROLE

1. Preheat the oven to 400°F and generously grease a 9 × 13-inch baking dish.

2. **SAUCE:** Bring the stock and ½ cup of the milk to a low boil in a saucepan. In a medium bowl, whisk the remaining ½ cup milk with the poultry seasoning and flour; add the mixture to the boiling liquid and whisk until a smooth creamy sauce forms.

3. **ASSEMBLY:** In a large bowl, mix the cream sauce with the quinoa, bacon, and ½ cup water and stir to combine. Pour the mixture into the prepared baking dish. Slice the chicken breasts into thin strips and lay the chicken strips over the top of the quinoa mixture. Sprinkle with the seasoning. Bake uncovered for 30 minutes.

4. **BROCCOLI:** While the casserole is in the oven, fill a sauté pan with an inch of water and bring to a boil. Place the broccoli in the boiling water for 1 minute, until it turns bright green. Drain into a colander and immediately run under cold water. Set aside.

5. **BAKE:** Remove the casserole from the oven, check the mixture by stirring it around in the dish, and if needed, bake for an additional 10 to 15 minutes

Serves 4

2 cups chicken stock

1 cup 2% milk

1 tsp. poultry seasoning

½ cup all-purpose flour

1 cup uncooked quinoa, rinsed

¼ cup cooked, crumbled turkey bacon

1 lb. boneless, skinless chicken breasts

2 tsp. seasoning (like Emeril's Essence or any basic blend you like)

3 cups fresh broccoli florets

¼ cup shredded Gruyère cheese

to get the right consistency. When the quinoa and chicken are cooked and the sauce is thickened, add the broccoli and a little bit of water (up to 1 cup) until the consistency is creamy and smooth and you can stir it up easily in the dish. Top with the cheese and bake just long enough to melt the cheese, about 5 minutes.

GRILLED LAMB CHOPS WITH WHEAT BERRY, STRAWBERRY, AND LACINATO KALE

1. Bring the stock and wheat berries to a boil in a medium saucepan over medium heat. Reduce the heat to low; cover and simmer until the berries are slightly chewy, about 22 minutes. Drain and rinse with cold water.

2. Heat a grill pan over medium-high heat for several minutes; then reduce the heat to medium. Sprinkle the lamb chops with 1 Tbsp. of the thyme, the curry powder, ½ tsp. of the salt, and ½ tsp. of the pepper.

3. Coat the grill pan with cooking spray. Place 6 lamb chops in the pan and grill to the desired doneness, about 5 minutes per side. Remove the chops from the pan and let stand for 5 minutes. Repeat with the remaining 6 chops.

4. Whisk the remaining ½ tsp. salt, ¼ tsp. pepper, and the oil, vinegar, shallots, and honey together in a large bowl.

5. Rub the sliced kale between your hands for several minutes or until slightly wilted. Add the wheat berries and kale to the vinegar mixture; toss to coat.

6. Top the salad with strawberries and cheese.

7. Divide the salad among 6 plates. Place the lamb chops on top of the salad.

Serves 6

6 cups beef or chicken stock

½ cup uncooked soft white wheat berries

12 4-oz. center-cut lamb loin chops

2 Tbsp. fresh thyme leaves

¾ tsp. curry powder

¾ tsp. sea salt

¾ tsp. freshly ground black pepper

Cooking spray

2 Tbsp. extra-virgin olive oil

1½ to 2 Tbsp. white balsamic vinegar

2 tsp. finely chopped shallots

¾ tsp. raw honey

1 bunch (8 oz.) of lacinato kale, thinly sliced, tough stems removed

1 cup sliced strawberries

1 oz. feta cheese, crumbled (¼ cup)

CAST-IRON STEAK DINNER WITH BUTTERY CAULIFLOWER MASH

1. Fit a large stockpot with a steamer basket, add 2 inches of water, and bring to a boil. Add the cauliflower florets, cover, and steam until very tender when pierced with a fork, 6 to 8 minutes. Set aside to cool for 4 to 5 minutes.

2. Put the garlic, milk, butter, garlic salt, ¼ tsp. pepper, and turmeric in a food processor along with the steamed cauliflower and process until smooth (you may need to do this in batches). Add a few tablespoons warm water if the mixture doesn't blend smoothly, to adjust the consistency. Transfer the mixture back to the stockpot to keep warm while you prepare the steak.

3. Preheat a cast-iron skillet over high heat until very hot, about 1 minute. Sprinkle the steak with salt and pepper. Put the oil in the skillet; then add the steak and cook, turning once or twice, until a sear forms and the meat is medium rare, 6 to 8 minutes. For a medium steak, cook 2 to 3 minutes more.

4. Transfer the steak to a cutting board and tent it lightly with aluminum foil. Let rest for 5 minutes. Serve with the cauliflower mash. (Green beans could also go well as an additional vegetable with the cauliflower.)

Serves 4

1 head cauliflower, cut into florets

4 garlic cloves, peeled and chopped

⅓ cup 2% milk

2 Tbsp. unsalted grass-fed butter

½ tsp. garlic salt

¼ tsp. freshly ground black pepper

¼ tsp. ground turmeric

4 8-oz. steaks such as strip or flat iron

Salt and freshly ground black pepper

1 Tbsp. extra-virgin olive oil

CHAPTER 13

TAKING THE WHEEL

We don't grow when things are easy; we grow when we face challenges. —Joyce Meyer

Well, there you have it. Everything you need is right in front of you. No more excuses. No more allowing doubts and fears to prevent you from achieving your goals. If you want to get in the best shape of your life, you now have the inspirational tools (a finely defined goal) and the practical tools (the exercise and meal plans) to make it a reality. For many of you, it could be the first time such crucial information has been made available to you. Make the most of it. Draw strength from the three *Ds*—be *Driven*, *Determined*, and *Disciplined*—and your body will indeed experience its own revolution.

But more than merely improving your waistline, carving your first six-pack, or adding slabs of lean muscle, I know that following the guidelines of this book will have a seismic impact on your overall well-being. I know that when you feel better, when you look better, when you're exhibiting the necessary dedication it takes to treat your body like it's a temple, the satisfaction and feeling of accomplishment permeate throughout every aspect of your life. Your mind, body, even your soul is enriched by the experience.

What is the soul exactly? It's a difficult question that requires a personal response.

For me, the soul is your true identity and functions as the basis for everything you do. It is not composed of mere hopes, wants, and wishes but is the honest core of who you are and what you're truly made of. It's not predetermined but formed and molded through experiences that have had an impact on your life. It will ultimately define what's important to you and whether you will accomplish that goal. All that I've encountered in my life—my time living in a U-Haul truck, meeting my wife, becoming a father, playing for the Packers, the people and projects I work with today—has affected my soul.

People don't wish to seek their soul because it's a pure reflection of truth. Most can't handle what they see. If the body and mind are weak, chances are the soul is conflicted—because the soul is your inner unconquerable giant that the mind and body learn to submit to and follow. That's why so many people who battle and succumb to overeating, or can't seem to find the right path to better health, go through life in pain. The disappointment and frustration that have evolved from their poor fitness have formed a cloud hovering over them that prevents their spirit from shining.

The power to complete any challenge in life lies within the soul. If your soul believes that nothing can beat you, nothing will. Failure or defeat may arise along the way, but it will only be temporary. If the mind exists to push the body, the soul is the muse for the mind. The three are interconnected and function at their fullest only when each link is strongest. If you make the commitment to eat, train, and live the lifestyle laid out in this book, if you're truly devoted to achieving a 3D Body Revolution, you will have that opportunity. That's why I wrote this book. All that's left for you to do is fight for what you want and make it a reality.

ACKNOWLEDGMENTS

I would like to express my gratitude to the many people who helped me see my love for fitness through to this book. To John Simon, Amy Goodson, Gina Mullen, Monica Henshaw, Jackie Burleson, and all those who provided support, read, wrote, offered comments, allowed me to quote their remarks, and assisted in the editing, proofreading, and design.

I would like to thank my writing partner, Jon Levey, for pushing and encouraging me to take a leap of faith.

Thanks to my publisher, Harmony Books.

Thanks to my good friend Brian Lammi. Without you this book would never have found its way to the hearts, minds, and souls of so many people.

Above all, I want to thank my wife, Betina Driver, and our children, Cristian, Christina, and Charity, who supported and encouraged me in spite of all the time it took me away from them. It was a long and exciting journey.

ABOUT THE AUTHOR

Donald Driver was a wide receiver for the Green Bay Packers NFL franchise, where he played from 1999 to 2012. He holds the all-time team records for receptions and receiving yards. He lives in Flower Mound, Texas, with his wife, Betina, and their son and two daughters. A role model on and off the field, Driver is a Super Bowl champion and a *Dancing with the Stars* winner. He has received multiple honors for his service to the community, including through the Donald Driver Foundation, which he started with his wife in 2004 to provide assistance for homeless mothers and underprivileged children.

DonaldDriver80.com